The Herbalist's Guide

The Herbalist's Guide

How to Build and Use Your Own Apothecary

MARY COLVIN, RH (AHG)

FOREWORD BY MIMI PRUNELLA HERNANDEZ, MS, RH (AHG)

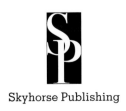

Skyhorse Publishing

Copyright © 2024 by Mary Colvin, RH (AHG)
Foreword copyright © 2024 by Mimi Prunella Hernandez, MS, RH (AHG)
Photography © 2024 by Mary Colvin unless otherwise noted

All rights reserved. No part of this book may be reproduced in any manner without the express written consent of the publisher, except in the case of brief excerpts in critical reviews or articles. All inquiries should be addressed to Skyhorse Publishing, 307 West 36th Street, 11th Floor, New York, NY 10018.

Skyhorse Publishing books may be purchased in bulk at special discounts for sales promotion, corporate gifts, fund-raising, or educational purposes. Special editions can also be created to specifications. For details, contact the Special Sales Department, Skyhorse Publishing, 307 West 36th Street, 11th Floor, New York, NY 10018 or info@skyhorsepublishing.com.

Skyhorse® and Skyhorse Publishing® are registered trademarks of Skyhorse Publishing, Inc.®, a Delaware corporation.

Visit our website at www.skyhorsepublishing.com.

10 9 8 7 6 5 4 3 2

Library of Congress Cataloging-in-Publication Data is available on file.

Cover design by Kai Texel
Cover photos by Mary Colvin, RH (AHG)

Print ISBN: 978-1-5107-7809-2
Ebook ISBN: 978-1-5107-7810-8

Printed in the United States of America

For my husband, Jack, as we celebrate our 25th wedding anniversary. Your support has been instrumental in where I am and in who I am today. You are the calm to my storm and a necessary part of my own well-being. I love you more than words can say.

For my three children, Melissa, Aaron, and Olivia. You have been raised on my concoctions, brews, and herbs while trusting me each time to make you feel better. I appreciate the trust and faith all three of you have unconditionally given me, and each of you have always been my inspiration and reason for continuing on this path. I am as proud of you as you are of me!

Contents

Foreword

The world of herbal medicine is vast and complex, and it can be overwhelming for those just starting out. That's why this book is such a valuable resource.

Mary is a remarkable professional who has dedicated her life to herbalism. As someone who has worked closely with Mary over the years in collaboration through the American Herbalists Guild and as an herbal colleague and confidant, I can attest to her passion for mentoring and dedication to helping others learn about the power of herbal medicine. One of the things I admire most about Mary is her ability to connect with people. Her knowledge of herbalism is vast, and she is always willing to share her expertise with others. She has a gift for teaching and has helped many people on their own path in herbalism. How clearly and beautifully her voice and teaching style come through in her writing is a wonder.

This book is a comprehensive guide to herbal medicine that is accessible to both beginners and experienced practitioners. It covers everything from the basics of herbalism to more advanced topics like creating herbal remedies and visioning steps toward a successful herbal practice. Mary's writing is clear and concise, providing plenty of practical advice and real-world exercises to help readers assimilate the material. Readers who engage in these exercises from start to finish will have a ready apothecary at hand upon completing this book.

One of the critical strengths of Mary's book is its focus on education. She emphasizes the importance of learning about plants and their properties from many perspectives, including from research and extending toward energetics. Mary provides a wealth of information on how to identify and harvest herbs, prepare them for use, and create effective herbal remedies. Throughout this book, she is right there with wholesome advice to the reader.

Another important aspect of Mary's book is its emphasis on building a personal apothecary, a collection of herbs, tinctures, and other remedies that an herbalist uses to support their family and community. Mary provides detailed instructions on creating your own apothecary, including tips on making effective tinctures and salves right from home. She also discusses the importance of ethical sourcing and sustainability, which is crucial for anyone working with plants.

Mary Colvin's book is a treasure for any budding herbalist; it is the exact book I wish I had when starting my own path in herbal medicine. Filled with practical advice and valuable tips, this book is a must-read for anyone interested in herbalism. Not only is it a guiding map for students, but it is also a valuable tool for teachers and mentors. Mary's knowledge, expertise, and passion for herbalism are genuinely inspiring, and I feel fortunate to celebrate the work of my friend and colleague.

—Mimi Prunella Hernandez, MS, RH (AHG)

Mimi Prunella Hernandez, RH (AHG), has dedicated her life to advocating for traditional and clinical herbal pathways. As an herbalist, she draws upon the influence of her Abuelitas and her background in biochemistry to weave together an herbal practice that's rooted in folk traditions and modern science. She is the author of *National Geographic Herbal* and the recipient of the American Botanical Council's 2023 Mark Blumenthal Herbal Community Builder Award. Mimi resides in the foothills of North Carolina, where she stewards the PonderLand, a native plant sanctuary that's part of the United Plant Savers Botanical Sanctuary Network. She was the executive director of the American Herbalists Guild from 2012 to 2023 and continues to work closely with this organization.

Introduction

I have been a lifetime admirer of plants, which began in the garden alongside my southern-raised maternal grandparents and my Sicilian paternal grandfather. I loved to dig my hands in the soft, fragrant loam and sit next to the towering pine trees for hours. Of course, I grew up in a time when you were sent outside to play until your mother finally called you inside for the night near dusk. I spent most of my childhood outdoors, and I have always felt a close connection to nature.

In 2006, I started experiencing excruciating shooting pains down my leg and debilitating lower back pain at only thirty-six years old. This pain prevented me from gardening, walking, sitting, and enjoying life with my husband and three children. I was finally diagnosed with degenerative and herniated L4 and L5 discs along with sciatic nerve pain. After suffering for a year and following all of the steps the doctors prescribed, I had to have surgery.

The surgery helped to stop the sciatica, but I continued having back pain. Eventually, I went back to the pain specialist only to be told that I would be in pain the rest of my life. The doctor explained that the fascia was damaged during the surgery procedure and that there was nothing more they could do except give me cortisone shots and prescribe pain pills. I was fed up with the dependency on pain pills to avoid pain, and the doctor's proclamation that I would not get any better, so I refused that diagnosis. I was a changed woman the moment I stood and declined the medicine they offered and walked out that door for the last time. I was determined to heal myself that day, and I have never regretted that decision. It was at this point that I chose to let the plants heal me, and I started my training in herbalism.

My training in herbalism consisted of formal education combined with years of self-study, mentorship, and clinical training. I am still learning something new every day. You never stop learning in herbalism. By 2018, I had enough training and experience to qualify as a Registered Herbalist with the American Herbalists Guild, and I eventually served as their treasurer and vice chair for a few years. I am currently running my own business as a clinical herbalist, formulator, mentor, author, and teacher.

I had formulated herbal formulas to help with my back pain, and the success at eliminating the pain and reclaiming my life caught the attention of a company called Eden's Answers. This company sold my formulas to the public beginning in 2012, and eventually sold their company in 2015 to Sprigs Life, Inc. I now have fifteen separate formulas being sold by Sprigs Life, and I enjoy a good business relationship with them to this day.

Training in herbalism has been, for me, an exciting journey of learning old traditions and different ways of incorporating nature into my family's life. At thirty-six, I would have never imagined how empowered I would feel with the life-changing knowledge I have obtained, or the success I would have in a new career. Training in herbalism includes a new understanding of the old ways, and a dedication to practicing the old ways in today's society. In a world where treating every symptom is more common than treating the cause, gaining this knowledge is important along with doing it safely and sustainably. How do we do that? It starts with traditional knowledge and combining that with the modern research and technologies of today.

This book will help you become more self-sufficient in herbalism, offer you training, and guide you in creating your own home apothecary. You will find purple boxes throughout this book that give you tips to make learning easier along with simple herbal recipes you can make at home. Visit www.herbalistmentor.com for more resources and extra training opportunities to help you expand in this field of study.

Follow the guided instructions throughout this book to create a fully functional apothecary. You will find this leaf symbol 🌿 after each herbal preparation to help you do just that. For those who live in an alcohol-free home, or those who want to avoid alcohol consumption altogether, skip the exercises making these types of herbal preparations.

By the end of this book, you will have the basic training, experience, and supplies to confidently make different herbal preparations to use in your own home. I hope to inspire you to continue your training into herbalism and move forward in your future studies. Welcome, and enjoy this journey!

PART ONE

Getting Started in Herbalism

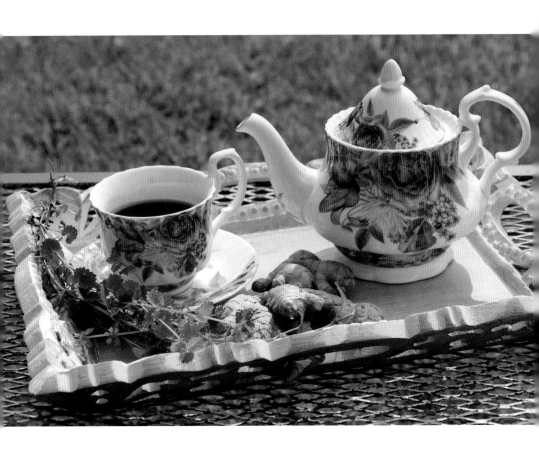

Chapter One
Herbalism

Herbalism is defined as the practice of using herbal medicine and using that knowledge to help the body heal, as well as contribute to the health of the individual using it. It is sometimes called herbal medicine, phytotherapy, medical herbalism, or botanical medicine. Herbology is the study of herbalism.

When I first started learning herbalism, I thought it was just a matter of learning about a few herbs and knowing how to make medicine with them. I quickly found out that there is much more to this field of study to learn. What became a fascination with herbs became a determination to learn more. Once I started this process, I couldn't stop. I was embarking on a journey to do what I am supposed to do, and working with the plants that make me happy. I also wanted to bring this happiness to others who feel the same passion. Sometimes an individual chooses to work with plants, and sometimes plants choose to work with an individual. Either way, the journey is fascinating and fulfilling.

Obviously, everyone needs to start with the basics of herbalism, but you can choose a variety of techniques, skills, and education to add on to this. This knowledge does not happen overnight, so give yourself permission to learn in steps. With today's technology, herbalism is inclusive to all that seek this traditional and modern knowledge. However, not everyone has the guidance they need. Plus, the amount of information that is available can be both contradicting and overwhelming. Without formal or traditional training, the self-taught individual is left to search for this knowledge themselves. There are many books on herbalism, but it is hard for that individual to know what steps they should follow in order to learn this information. They need personal guidance on the sequence of learning so that they can understand the information given to them before moving on. If you were this individual in the past, or are wanting guidance right now with learning herbalism, you are in the right place.

Learning herbalism is a skill that everyone should have, even if it's just the basics. You can stock your own herbal apothecary at home and help to support your family or friends as needed with just a few well-chosen herbs. The school I attended taught how to use one hundred herbs over a period of two years, but this can be overwhelming. I think I did my best working with ten herbs at a time in many different ways. You don't need to know them all right away—just a few very well.

What does the study of herbal medicine include? How does this knowledge help the body heal? What does it mean to contribute to the health of the individual using it? Let's talk about that right now.

The study of herbal medicine includes knowing how to identify, harvest, process, and dose herbs. Learning botany is a definite bonus in this field and a skill that will benefit you later if you come across plants that you do not know. It also includes knowing the different medicinal actions herbs provide for the body, getting to know and understand the taste and how those can affect the body, how to balance the correct herb with the person needing it, and what dose each person will need. It takes some time to learn the terms used in herbalism. Start by memorizing the terms, researching the herbs thoroughly, then tasting and experiencing the herbs to understand how each of their properties and actions work

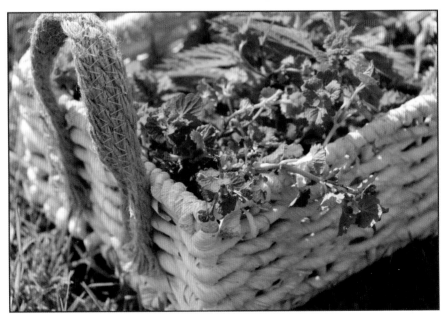

Basket of ground ivy (*Glechoma hederacea*)

with the body. You read about herbs, but it will never be the same as experiencing the herbs personally. Combining this knowledge will benefit you in helping others in a variety of situations.

Those who study herbalism come from many different cultures, backgrounds, and locations. All of this will help you to determine what kind of herbalist you wish to be—how you practice, what herbs are available, what traditions you follow, and what modalities you include in your healing practices. There are also multiple medical systems within herbalism that you can choose to study.

Think about your own culture and upbringing and how this could affect your beliefs, your way of living, your traditions in your family and community, and how you wish herbalism to fit into your life. Every person will have a different path in herbalism and a different way of practicing and that is perfectly fine. Herbalists do not fit in a one-size-fits-all category—they have different philosophies, different religions, different herbs located within their community, and different ways of living. Accordingly, this book is not for any one specific type of herbalist. It is meant for all to take in the information, research on their own, experience herbalism, build their apothecary, and incorporate their own healing philosophies and traditions into their practice that feels comfortable to them.

My oldest daughter wanted an herbal first aid kit to take with her to college. She was raised for a good part of her life on Western herbalism as I was learning and practicing. She knows firsthand how herbs can help and has a basic knowledge of them. I consider her an herbalist even though she isn't an expert or wants to continue her study in this area. She knows a few herbs very well, as well as how and when to use them. She became the resident herbalist herself in her college dorm when other students were in need. When she came home, we restocked her supply kit and she would tell me how the students appreciated her help. As she begins raising her own family, she will once again bring into her life the herbs she is familiar with. She might not fit the traditional label of herbalist, but she definitely is one. She can continue her learning in the future, or just stick with what she knows right now.

How does the study of herbs help the body heal? I will be discussing medicinal properties (sometimes called medicinal actions) and energetics in this book that will help more in this understanding. To be honest with you, society is just beginning to understand "how" an herb works on the body with modern scientific research. Traditionally, herbalists and physicians of old used experience, intuition, and observation knowing that an herb worked without needing to know how it worked. It just did. This knowledge was passed down through the generations and between different cultures.

Saint-John's-wort (*Hypericum perfoliatum*) was traditionally used as wound medicine in medieval times and worked consistently way before what we recognize as modern science even came into existence. Science can, however, be useful in finding other nontraditional ways an herb can be beneficial, such as how an herb/constituent interacts with pharmaceuticals or the process/path an herb takes in the body. There can be a balance consisting of both traditional and modern medicine. This is where your foundation as an herbalist can be chosen. Some herbalists only work with herbs based on proven scientific studies, or only trust traditional knowledge that has been used for centuries. Other herbalists combine both approaches in their practice. I am one of those "other" herbalists. So, the answer to the question "how do herbs help the body heal?" depends on your attitude toward traditional knowledge and scientific studies along with learning the actions and energetics of herbalism.

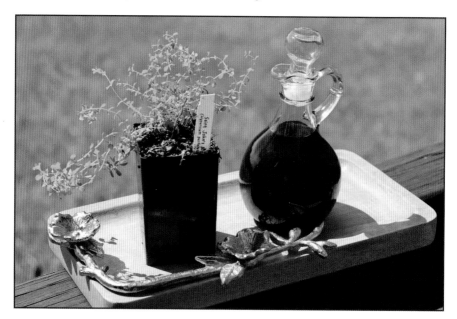

Oil infused with Saint-John's-wort

Contributing to the health of an individual refers to choosing the right herb(s) or having the right recommendations for each individual specifically. Herbs are sometimes categorized in terms of a specific condition that they address, but we need to choose an herb that works best for the person needing it. An example I like to give is ginger (*Zingiber officinale*) being recommended for nausea. Have you ever known someone who has tried ginger and it made the nausea or other symptoms worse, or they don't like using it? Ginger is energetically a very warming and drying herb. For an individual who has heat already in their system, or has a warm or dry constitution, this herb is not necessarily for them. It could either aggravate the symptoms or cause other disagreements within the individual. These individuals would be better off with a cooling anti-nausea herb such as raspberry (*Rubus idaeus*) leaves in order to counter the heat in their body while reducing the nausea. Think of this as a balancing act between the correct herbal action and the bodily needs of each individual.

Contributing to the health of an individual also means that herbs are only a portion of how an individual reaches health. The opposite of health is disease, and returning to health involves more than just using herbs. Nutrition, lifestyle changes, counseling, and other healing methods might be used alongside herbs in order for the body to start healing. Contributing to the health of an individual also includes doing no harm to that person. It is important that you keep safety in your mind at all times. This includes knowing the contraindications and interactions of each herb based on the conditions the individual might have, and pharmaceutical medications that they are taking. I recommend learning this information before using an herb. It also means using these herbs in a traditional and respectful way. Herbalists do not inject herbs directly into the bloodstream or use herbs/doses that they know will harm a person. Just because herbs are natural doesn't mean they are always safe. Some herbs are harmful in larger doses too. This is where training and research come in prior to the use of an herb.

I believe that there should be more well-trained herbalists to contribute their skills in their communities or, at the very least, someone in every home that understands the basics. Herbalism can work alongside modern medicine, or even be a first step before following up with modern medicine. I am not against doctors, surgery, pharmaceuticals, or hospitalization. However, I believe that we can benefit from taking responsibility for our own health first in a nonemergency situation.

Mary's Advice

Not all herbalists grow their own herbs, prepare their own medicine, sell their formulas, make a career out of it, or consult with clients. If you want to use herbs in your own home just for your family and friends, that is okay. You don't have to do it all. You can also purchase herbal medicine elsewhere from sustainable and reputable resources.

An increase in the number of herbalists could help to lower the costs of health care and health insurance in the long run. This same increase could also drive the costs of herbs and supplements upward and contribute to the overharvesting of certain herbs if all herbalists refrain from growing/harvesting their own herbs sustainably. I think an important job we all have as herbalists is to teach sustainable harvesting and educate others on how to grow herbs themselves if possible. Not every household has the space to grow large gardens, but as communities we can help to sustain gardening through container gardening, community gardens, and more. We can also come together and start new businesses growing herbs and selling them to our communities.

Not every herbalist needs to be a clinical herbalist like me. There is a huge need for growers to provide these resources so that our wild herbs are not overharvested to extinction and more of the public has access to these plants for medicine. The need for teachers, however, in both growing and using herbs is an absolute necessity. As you continue to learn about herbalism, consider taking on the responsibility of learning new gardening skills or techniques, growing new or at-risk herbs, and passing your knowledge on to others.

I want to emphasize that herbalists do not use herbs as a replacement for pharmaceuticals, nor do they use an herb for a specific disease. Herbs do not work the same way as pharmaceuticals, and an herb for arthritis does not exist. Most diseases need additional lifestyle changes that an herb alone will not fix.

Chapter Two
Individual and Scientific Research

Understanding where you are getting your information about herbalism is just as important as what information you are getting. There can be a lot of conflicting, confusing, and misleading information out there. As a student studying on your own, it is up to you to continue researching from the right resources to get the correct and most reliable information. There are two different kinds of research in herbalism that I am referring to. One is individual research where the student is looking up information, and the other is scientific research where the scientists are trying to find and prove answers. One has red flags that you should be aware of that will help you in your research of information, and the other has some points to consider to understand how their information was obtained. After reading about each herb in this book, you will be asked to research them in further detail prior to working with each in a hands-on exercise. This chapter will help with that process.

Starting with individual research, there are multiple places to find the information you are looking for. Books, the internet, classes, conferences, organizations, and individual teachers are just some of the different resources to study from. In order to better understand the thirty-five herbs in this book, you will need to know their medicinal properties, traditional and modern uses, the best menstruum to extract the medicine from, the potential contraindications and interactions associated with them, their growing conditions, if they are considered at-risk, and much more.

It's easy to do an online search for this information, but how do you know who or what to believe? The best way to maneuver through all this information is to have some guidelines to follow. My guidelines consist of the following:

- Research at least ten different resources. Don't just watch one video on how an herb can benefit you or learn from just one herbalist on how they use that herb. You will have more insights and beneficial information by learning from both the past and present in your research and from multiple people. Never take the word of one person or one school and believe it's the gospel. This includes me! I want you to do your own research and come to the best conclusion for you and your apothecary.
- Research each one of your resources! There are a lot of herbalists on the internet telling people how to practice herbalism, but this information is sometimes incorrect and can be dangerous. The intent isn't always to deceive or cause harm, but if they are beginner herbalists themselves, they shouldn't be teaching others. The same goes for someone using credentials to further their credibility with herbs. Being a doctor does not mean that a person is trained or experienced using whole herbs. Many like to use supplements if they even do that. You need to understand the difference. Here's more to consider:
  - Look for their experience practicing herbalism (more than a few years).
  - Look for any mention of their own training, mentors, or schooling. Investigate each one of these. Do their credentials pertain to herbalism? Look for reviews of individuals or schools if applicable along with the length of training offered and the subjects taught. (A beginner course is not enough training in herbalism to be teaching others.)
  - Look for clinical training, clinical experience, and clinical hours with clients that they have had. (Talking to customers in a health food store is not equivalent to this kind of training and experience.)
- Look for red flags. These could be words they use or the lack of information that they give. You want to be wary of information given if any of these points apply:
  - Not mentioning their own experience.
  - Not mentioning where they were trained and/or not giving credit to those who have trained or mentored them.
  - An individual herbalist who sells products without mentioning the two points above. Whenever I run across a website or link, I

personally look for an "about the herbalist" section. If it's not there, I move on.

- As an unlicensed practitioner, they are saying or using the words *cure*, *treat*, *diagnose*, or *this herb is a natural* "insert pharmaceutical medicine here." One example is where someone might say they have experienced an herbal cure for themselves, and it will cure everyone else too. Any of these words or sayings can be dangerous to the herbal community as a whole. I see this often on social media, and it is a big red flag for me.

- Saying "everyone should or could take this herb." This is something a trained herbalist would not say because everyone has different constitutions, conditions, medications, or health that affects whether or not they can take the herb, or whether the herb will benefit them if at all.

- They are using the wrong terminology. This is why it's so important for you to know the correct terminology. You want to be able to spot untrained herbalists, and you don't want to be considered one from this category in the future. One that I see often is when someone says all herbal extracts are called tinctures. This is an untrue statement, and as you continue to read this book, you will understand why.

- Thoroughly check all information you receive from reliable resources. Social media and Google by themselves are not always reliable resources. Take what you read with a grain of salt until you find multiple reliable resources to confirm it. Go back to the first two points in this list!

- Continue learning. Information can change, techniques can improve, you could learn information you didn't realize, or you could see another person's viewpoint. Learning is continuous in herbalism.

When it comes to researching scientific studies, there are some things you need to be aware of. First, most research is funded for a purpose, and it could benefit different people. Whether herbs are being studied to develop a new pharmaceutical medicine, provide safety information, etc., knowing who is funding the study and the purpose of each one is important information to consider. Here are some other points that you might consider to fully understand a study:

- The way the herb is being observed or studied. Is the herb being tested in a test tube or petri dish (in vitro), or done on a living organism (in vivo)?
- If they are in vivo studies, are they being studied on animals or humans?
- If humans, how many participants?
- How long was the study observed?
- How is the herb prepared? Is an extract used, or an isolated constituent?
- How is the herb delivered? Is it injected, used topically, or taken internally?
- Where was the study published?
- Is the publication peer-reviewed?

These are just some questions that you want to investigate or understand as you are looking at a scientific study about an herb, its benefits and uses, or its suggested dangers. Not all of these questions will pertain to a single study. It's possible for a study to be looking at the types of constituents an herb has or its pharmacological uses to study further in the future. Just like your individual research, get your scientific research from multiple sources. It is best that they are peer-reviewed and studied the way herbalism is practiced with clinical trials consisting of numerous human participants and a lengthy observation time. Of course, this would be a best-case scenario when it comes to researching herbalism, but not always probable, as not all studies are observed this way. Just something to keep in the back of your mind as you are researching information.

The best advice I can give about researching information about herbalism is to check multiple types of resources, verify experience and credentials from these resources, and use information from both the past and the present. Do not limit yourself to just one type of resource either! This will ensure that you have different views, techniques of practicing, reliable safety information, and dependable information to base your knowledge on. Use this chapter as a reference when needed.

Chapter Three
Categories of Herbalism

Herbalism incorporates the use of many different parts of the plant, utilizing whole plant material in herbal preparations to extract multiple constituents, minerals, or vitamins for medicine or nutrition. These subcategories use only one part of the plant, use only one constituent, have a different philosophy altogether, or only have one way to administer their effects. Each of these subcategories has benefits and is great to learn once you are trained in herbalism itself.

Essential Oils

Essential oils are the isolated and condensed volatile oils (aroma component) of an herb and are used in aromatherapy. Aromatherapy utilizes the medicinal actions of these volatile oils through scent. They are also added to oil-based salves or ointments to use externally for scent or medicinal purposes. Essential oils are not herbs, but just one type of constituent among many contained within a plant. Either the leaves or the flowers go through a process called steam distillation, which isolates these volatile oils. It takes large amounts of plant material to condense just a small ounce of essential oil.

Essential oils are not to be confused with infused oils, which are plant materials (leaves, flowers, bark, or roots) infused into a base oil such as olive, jojoba, sweet almond, etc. These infused oils create an oil, ointment, or salve for healing wounds, rashes, muscle aches, etc.

Essential oils have antibacterial, antiviral, antifungal, nervine, and antispasmodic properties. You will get these same properties from the plant the volatile oils originated from as well. What you won't get from essential oils are the many other constituents that you can extract from a plant. An example is peppermint essential oil. You can use this oil for spasms and headaches from tension, but you will not receive the astringency benefits this plant can give you because the tannins are not contained in the volatile oil. Peppermint as a whole plant has more medicinal uses than the isolated essential oil alone.

There is a lot of misinformation among the general public about the correct use and safety of essential oils. Some multilevel marketing businesses encourage customers to use their essential oils internally, but many essential oils should not be ingested. Even when internal ingestion is appropriate, they should only be ingested under the supervision of a clinical aromatherapist or other professionally trained practitioner. A multilevel marketing representative who recommends internal ingestion of essential oils does not necessarily have the correct training in clinical herbalism or clinical aromatherapy. Since essential oils are derived from herbs, it is important for everyone to learn about herbalism first. When working with herbs, it is very important to know and understand these seven points:

1. How the herb contributes to healing (the medicinal actions on the body).
2. What part of the plant should be used.
3. How best to extract the action needed.
4. How the herb interacts with medications.
5. How the herb contraindicates with certain conditions.
6. How to apply or administer the herb.
7. The correct dosage.

These same points need to be understood and considered when working with essential oils because they are a part of an herb. Essential oils produce actions, interact with medications, have contraindications, have certain applications, and have maximum permissible percentages (dermal limits) that must be adhered to. Safety is a big component of herbalism, and harmful effects should always be considered first. Using essential oils internally or not diluting them before application can be particularly harmful to individuals with certain conditions or who take certain pharmaceutical medications. If not seen immediately, the effects can accumulate and cause further issues down the road. If an individual needs to take an herb internally, I recommend incorporating it into the diet, or taking an herbal preparation made with it after thoroughly researching the herb for safety first. I utilize essential oils for aromatherapy and add them to my oil-infused herbal preparations for scent or medicinal actions when needed.

Since large amounts of plant material are needed to make a small bottle of essential oil, they can contribute to the overharvesting of certain plants. It is best to use smaller amounts when needed for aromatherapy, and the whole herb for other medicinal uses. Less plant material of the herb is needed to create a tea, tincture, or other herbal preparation at home.

Exercise

Research both lavender and rosemary and compare medicinal properties and types of constituents they contain, safety, contraindications and interactions, overall costs, and the different ways each should be used. This will give you a good idea of the differences between the two.

Make a simple external spray oil for tension. Pick an oil of your choosing and pour into a four-ounce glass spray bottle. Add sixteen drops each of lavender and rosemary essential oils. Mix thoroughly, spray across the back of the shoulders, and rub the oil into the skin. Spray on the wrists to enjoy the aromatherapy too!

🌿 *Add this healing aromatic oil to your apothecary!*

Homeopathy

When I tell someone that I am an herbalist, they sometimes confuse that term with homeopathy. There are some similarities between the two, but mostly differences. Herbalism's philosophy is about creating a homeostasis within the body and balancing the herbs with the individual, and homeopathy's philosophy is "like curing like." It follows the law of similars, which holds that a medicinal agent causes the same symptoms that it cures. The homeopath sets out to find the similarity between the symptoms produced by the disease and those produced by the medicine.[1] Homeopathy can use plants, minerals, animal, or chemical substances in diluted amounts to remedy symptoms of a disease that in larger amounts they could cause.

Apart from the philosophy, homeopathy also differs from herbalism in the amount of medicine contained in the remedy. Homeopathic medicine is diluted and delivered in such a minute amount to prevent negative side effects. However, the World Health Organization states:

> Still, there are a few aspects of the production of homeopathic medicines that could constitute potential safety hazards. Firstly, not all homeopathic medicines are administered at a high dilution. Sometimes, a homeopathic medicine made from source material, such as a mother tincture, is administered in the most concentrated form. Secondly, homeopathic medicines are made from a wide range of natural or synthetic sources: minerals and chemicals, but also plant materials, including roots, stems, leaves, flowers, bark, pollen, lichen, moss, ferns, and algae; microorganisms, including fungi, bacteria, viruses, and plant parasites; animal organs, tissues, secretions, and cell lines. Human materials may include tissues, secretions, hormones, and cell lines. Some of these source materials constitute potential safety hazards, even at high dilutions.[2]

I believe the confusion between herbalism and homeopathy is because both forms of healing use whole plants, and the general public is not familiar with the particulars of each. Even with these differences, homeopathy can be considered a category of herbalism based on its healing aspects using plants, but it is also its own separate form of alternative healing.

Exercise

Find a homeopathic product and research the herbs it contains. Find out what this product is used for. Would these same plants be utilized in herbalism in the same way? If so, how? If not, why?

Flower Essences

If you have heard of Bach Flower Remedies or Australian Bush Flower Essences, you are familiar with the concept of flower essences. For those who are not or who haven't heard of either brand, flower essences are used for healing the emotional level of an individual. They are prepared using fresh flowers extracted in pure water by the sun. The final product is combined with brandy for more stability or shelf-life. I believe all herbs can work on the emotional level, but flower essences are for those who need even more focus on emotional healing. I have heard some people refer to flower essences as "vibrational medicine."

Mary's Advice

Decide which flowers you want to make into a flower essence. Create a calendar for each flower's bloom time and follow this schedule throughout the growing season. Make the flower essences according to your calendar, then research the benefits of each before using. Add these flower essences to your home apothecary.

Dr. Edward Bach (1886–1936) developed these flower remedies through his work in homeopathy in the 1930s. Even though great herbalists in the past offered herbal medicine as a means of cheering, consoling, quieting, uplifting, and settling the mind and the emotions, Dr. Bach made a connection between feelings and actual physical illness.[3] These flower remedies were his answer to confronting disease.

You can make your own flower essences by first adding pure spring or well water to a clean bowl, then either laying flowers flat on top of

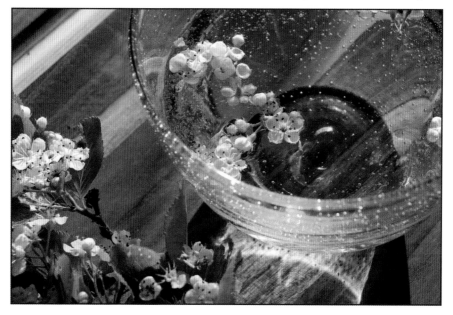

Creating hawthorn flower essence

the water or adding flowers to another container and submerging this container in the water bowl. Place the bowl in full sun. Once the flowers begin to wilt (within an hour or so), strain the water and fill a bottle equaling 50:50 of the infused water and brandy. This is considered the "mother tincture." I make my stock bottles by combining half the bottle with the mother tincture and the other half with brandy. I then use this diluted mother tincture to make individual dosage bottles for my clients. Dosage bottles are made by taking two to ten drops of the stock bottle, and combining it in a one-ounce bottle with half spring water and half brandy. The individual typically takes four drops under the tongue three times daily. This has worked really well for me and my clients.

Flower essences are similar to homeopathy in that they are greatly diluted, but they do not follow the "like curing like" philosophy of homeopathy. Just as I consider homeopathy a category of herbalism even though it could be its own form of alternative healing, I consider flower essences a category of herbalism because they use flowers and because their use combines well with herbalism.

Exercise

In the spring, summer, and autumn, choose flowers growing near you that you are drawn to and make a flower essence with them. Follow the directions above to make one or more for your own use. Store these flower essences in dark bottles in a cool, dark cupboard. Label each mother tincture with the flower name and the word "mother" and do the same for the stock bottles with the flower name and the word "stock." Use the stock bottles to create dosage bottles, then use the mother tincture to refill the stock bottles. Keep a journal with the names of the different flower essences you have along with a description of how that flower can help.

🍃 *Congratulations! You just added flower essences to your apothecary!*

Chapter Four
The Apothecary

The apothecary was once a place or person where herbs, spices, and herbal preparations were made and provided to customers. They also provided other products consisting of cosmetics, perfumes, dyes, and skin care. The term apothecary is an older term that refers to the selling of medicine that involves a multitude of other resources rather than just herbs. This term is still used today, but it is steeped with legal implications that I will explain at the end of this chapter. The profession dates back to 2600 BC to ancient Babylon, where we find clay tablets with medical texts recording symptoms, the prescriptions, and the directions for compounding it.

The apothecary was originally part of the grocery business, but the official Worshipful Society of Apothecaries, established in 1617, separated apothecaries from groceries. In medieval times, the apothecary provided medicine for the common people. Trained physicians were usually too expensive, and the customer could either grow and make their own medicine, go to a monastery, or visit a local apothecary.[4] The apothecary was trained in the use of herbs and other sources along with the anatomy of the body to provide advice and services to their customers. They used knowledge of the individual and the illness to prepare the correct medicine for them. This is similar to the job description of a clinical herbalist working with herbs today.

Apothecaries were also known as "spicers" or "pepperers" due to their work weighing out herbs and spices. They were involved in importation and distribution of spices for cooking or in the preparation of other products such as spiced wine. When the apothecary was first established, they started growing their own herbs to sell. Eventually, supply chains developed to stock their inventory. Some medicine was prepared ahead of time and stocked on the shelves to sell to the public much as a pharmacy would today.[5]

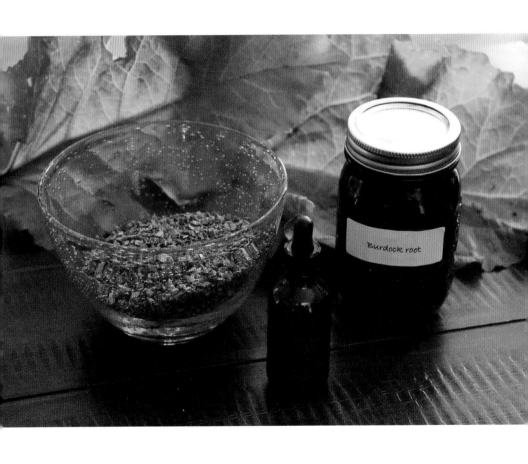

After that basic introduction, I want to discuss legal implications surrounding the term "apothecary." Most people understand that an apothecary involves using herbs for medicine and skin care and would never confuse it with today's drugstore or pharmacy. "Apothecary" is an archaic term that drugstores and pharmacies do not utilize today, yet they are claiming the name just the same in common law. In the state of Ohio where I reside, Ohio Revised Code states:

> No place except a pharmacy licensed as a terminal distributor of dangerous drugs and no person except a licensed pharmacist shall display any sign or advertise in any fashion using the words "pharmacy, "drugs," "drugstore," "drug-store supplies," "pharmacist," "druggist," "pharmaceutical chemist," "apothecary," "drug sundries," "medicine," or any of these words or their equivalent, in any manner.[6]

All of these terms relate to medicine, pharmacy, or drugs except apothecary. The Ohio state government claims that apothecaries are associated with pharmaceutical medicine, yet herbal medicine differs from the modern medicine of today. That is, of course, unless an herb such as marijuana is regulated by the state and prescribed by a doctor to be distributed by licensed facilities. It belies common sense, but it appeals to the regulating body, licensed professionals, and pharmaceutical providers.

All that being said, I use the word apothecary in this book to refer to herbal medicine being made in your own home for your family and friends. If you choose to sell herbal medicine, herbs, or products containing herbs, be sure to look up your own state laws. There will be more information and resources for you at the end of this book about the legal challenges when selling to the public.

Chapter Five
Herbalism and Botany

Within the study of herbalism, it is very beneficial and important to understand botany and botanical terms. Botany is the study of all plant life including their structure, environment, and how they survive. It is necessary to know these parts of the plant in order to distinguish identification patterns. Why is this needed in herbalism? You want to make sure you are 100 percent correct in the identification of an herb or plant before harvesting, making medicine with it, and finally consuming the product. Botany skills can also help identify plants unknown to you. Once you feel more confident in your skills to identify plants, you will become more confident in yourself as an herbalist.

When I was a child, I wanted to be a botanist or horticulturist. Unfortunately, finances kept me from achieving my goal, but it did not stop me from pursuing the knowledge on my own. I learned a lot about growing plants from my family and two years in college at Ohio State University. I had basic botany, greenhouse operations, and herbaceous plant courses in college, but I wanted to learn more. I found botany so interesting because a plant can tell you a story about itself by studying its location, soil composition, adaptability to certain situations, and who its neighbors are. You need to use your senses to recognize these stories, and between your senses and knowledge, learn to interpret them.

Mary's Advice

Learn the Latin name of an herb or plant and study the botanical terms associated with it to better understand its identifying features.

Just as botanical terms are beneficial in herbalism, so is Latin. Latin is considered a dead language, but because it cannot evolve, it is useful for naming plants. You are not required to know how to speak, write, or interpret Latin. You just need to know Latin names when identifying your plants. There are hundreds of different viburnum species growing

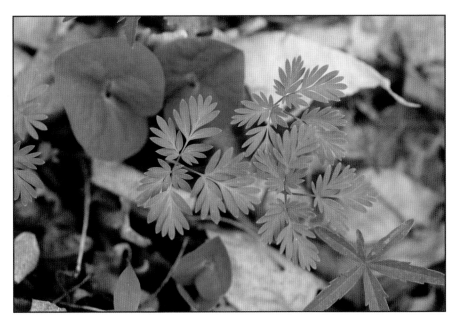

Woodland leaf shapes

in the United States. How do you know which one you have in your backyard? You would need to notice the parts of the shrub, including leaf shape, margins, flower petals, bark, or other distinguishing aspects of the plant's environment to correctly identify it. The other reason Latin names are so important is that they help distinguish one plant from another, which is why each species has its own Latin name. It would cause confusion if you were personally telling someone to grow lungwort, which is a common name for multiple herbs benefiting the lungs. The word "wort" means herb, and folklore can have many of the same common names, especially in different localities. This is why it is important to know scientific names when you are talking about growing or using an herb for medicinal purposes.

When you are researching a plant, you will find information about its classification. The most important classifications I look for are family, genus, and species. Each plant is classified by its traits and patterns into a certain family and separated further by genus and species within that family.

When you are writing or reading about more than one herb in a genus, the first genus and species are written out, and the second genus is abbreviated with the species spelled out. An example would be

Arctium lappa and *A. minus*. This example is speaking about two burdock species used to make medicine in the genus *Arctium*. If you are repeating *Arctium lappa* in the same document, you would spell out the genus first, then abbreviate afterward. This prevents the need to keep spelling out the same genus multiple times.

Knowing the Latin names of plants can also help you determine if plants are interchangeable in a genus. If a genus is followed by spp., that would mean all species are interchangeable medicinally. An example would be goldenrod (*Solidago* spp.).

Mary's Advice

I learned so much about plant families from a book called *Botany in a Day* by Thomas J. Elpel. This would be a great resource to help you understand plant families, their identification, common constituents, and common medicinal properties.

Knowing about the patterns of plant families is another beneficial skill in herbalism that can help you identify not only a plant, but also the type of constituents in that plant and its common medicinal properties. When I am out in the woods and come upon a plant I do not know, I first look for signs or patterns of the family. Once that is established, I then proceed with documenting the leaf shape, margins, flowers, veining patterns, and more. I usually take a camera with me on my explorations and a journal to write down these findings. I document when the plant is growing, what type of area it's located in, what type of soil it resides in, what other plants are around it, and where exactly I found it. I then take all of this information and research for the correct species identification. It is not always easy to do this, but practice makes perfect.

This type of information could help you become a better herbalist, especially if you want to document herbs in your area, conduct herb identification walks for your community, or identify plants for others. However, it is not necessary to know anything more in botany than the Latin names of plants and the plant families as an herbalist, especially if you do not plan to participate in the aforementioned activities or harvest in the wild.

Exercise

Pick any herb you would like to research. Are there other herbs in the world with the same common name? What is the Latin name, and what does it mean? How is this plant classified, and why? Pick a couple other herbs in the same family and learn their Latin names as well. What are the similar botanical patterns? Do these herbs have similar medicinal properties? Do these herbs grow in the same area as your original herb? Continue researching these herbs for more information.

PART TWO
Harvesting Basics

Chapter Six
Harvesting Rules

Every person considering harvesting from the wild needs to understand the following harvesting rules. These honorary rules are standard practice for all the herbalists that care about the continuation of medicinal herbs. Before harvesting in the wild, familiarize yourself with identification terms and practice looking for them. When teaching about herbalism, hosting herb walks, or showing others how to harvest herbs, it is good to teach these rules in order to avoid overharvesting. It is our duty as stewards to these plants to do this.

> ### Mary's Advice
> When you are hiking or taking a walk, remember to document in your journal where a plant is located to see if the plant comes back year after year.

I have heard horror stories from other herbalists that have shown some of their students a group of plants that can be used as medicine only to return later and find them all gone. The students were not taught the basic rules and they most likely didn't know any better, but the damage was already done. We need to keep in mind that these plants are not placed here just for our nutritive and medicinal uses. Animals, insects, birds, and the entire ecosystem are affected by their absence. Some people see dollar signs when they come upon a large patch of herbs, but that is never a good reason to take them all. Please take some time to know these harvesting rules and follow the guidelines they represent so that future generations can know, appreciate, and benefit from these plants as well.

1. **Be 100 percent clear on the identification of the plant before proceeding to harvest.** Mistakes can be made and there are plant similarities such as flower shapes, similar leaf patterns, and colored berries

that could cause confusion when harvesting. Know your plant thoroughly before harvesting.

2. **Only harvest what you need.** This prevents overharvesting and the waste of an herb. Start with just enough to prepare each medicine you need in your apothecary and have some extra stored for use through the rest of the year. As you work with different herbal preparations, you will have a better estimate of how much is needed for each and how much you need for your family or business.

3. **Harvest only ⅓ of the plant.** This guideline prevents damage to the plant and ensures the continuation of its species. If you take more than a third of the plant itself, the plant could die.

4. **Only harvest ⅓ of a group of plants.** This guideline prevents the depletion of a certain herb in an area. You might think you have hit the jackpot when you finally find that one herb you have been looking all over for, but you should pass it up and find a larger patch where you will have an opportunity to harvest sustainably. At this point, harvest a third of the population and leave the remaining ⅔ to keep them reproducing and spreading in the wild. By following this rule, you will have some next year and the remaining years for harvesting. Always take the time to look for more of an herb in the wild or grow some yourself to save the wild population.

5. **Learn to harvest correctly.** This guideline prevents damage to the plant. An example is harvesting bark. If you cut the bark in a circumference around the tree (girdling), the tree can die.

6. **Harvest at the correct time.** When harvesting roots of plants, make sure that the seeds are ready to disperse and be replanted in the fall. It is up to the individual harvesting to replant these seeds. This ensures the survival of that species.

7. **Always ask permission to harvest on land that is not yours.** This is common courtesy and helps to avoid any legal or insurance issues.

8. **Never harvest from government-owned land!** Government-owned lands have the sole purpose of protecting the very plants you want to harvest for future generations. They are also there for many other taxpayers to enjoy visually and contribute to the ecosystem they belong to. You may contact the office or the conservationist on duty to ask permission, or for them to personally accompany you. They are

usually very accommodating if you want to harvest invasive plants or what they might consider a weed. I have personally contacted local parks about harvesting burdock roots, which they were happy to oblige as long as someone from their office was with me. However, they are less receptive if there are small numbers of plants on the land or a plant is at-risk. All of these rules serve a purpose, and that is to protect plants and our ecosystem, which all of us in this field should appreciate and adhere to.

Exercise

Take a walk out in nature and notice how plants are growing. Are they growing as single plants placed here and there or in large patches? How many can you find of one species? Choose one plant growing in the wild and see if you can find more. Should you be harvesting from this plant? Is it a common plant in your area or do you need to go elsewhere to find it? Should you grow it yourself?

Chapter Seven
Sustainability Issues

Today, we have the largest population of people living on this planet. More land and forests are being torn down and replaced with homes, businesses, parking lots, or infrastructure. Our trash is filling up landfills and littering the ocean. This can cause a myriad of issues including the extinction of different species of animals, insects, birds, and plants. We might not be individually responsible for this happening, but all of us together have a responsibility to fight for change. We can make personal choices in our lives that individually might not seem like enough but could make a huge impact in greater forces.

Many of these choices could be in the form of choosing recyclable over nonrecyclable materials (paper over plastic, reusable bags over plastic bags, or glass storage containers over plastic ones). Each of us can do what we can to make a difference if we choose to. Sustainability to

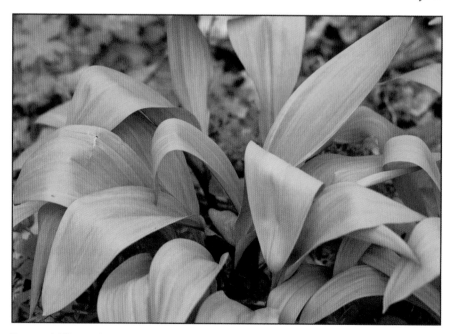

Ramps (*Allium tricoccum*)

me is the avoidance of depleting our natural resources and contributing to the balance of the ecosystem. As herbalists, we are focused on the survival of our plants for future generations, but we should also consider the sustainability of our planet too. What can we personally do to make a difference? What can we do to contribute to the well-being of our planet? What choices could we make to sustain our plant medicine and show that we can take a part in the future survival of these plants? These are questions we should be asking ourselves especially when we are contributing to the harvesting of these plants and using their resources.

Following the harvesting rules from the last chapter is a good start in helping plant populations flourish, but there is more we can do.

1. **Know what native plants in your area are at-risk.** You can stay updated about native plants by visiting the United Plant Savers website at www.unitedplantsavers.org. Their mission is to protect native medicinal plants of the United States and Canada while ensuring an abundant renewable supply of medicinal plants for generations to come. When you become a member, you receive the annual *Journal of Medicinal Plant Conservation* as well as other benefits. This information is important to know so you aren't contributing to the demise of these plants for the future. United Plant Savers also educate the public on how they can help in the continuation of these at-risk herbs.

2. **Plant at-risk herbs.** Please try planting these herbs yourself if you have the space, land, or know someone that does. Be sure to ask permission to plant on someone else's land. Learn about the growing conditions of these plants as well so that they can flourish.

3. **Buy your herbs from reputable sources.** Before you buy from someone, ask them if they follow sustainable harvesting practices. They should be able to tell you where they purchase their bulk herbs from, if they are non-GMO or organic, or if they donate to the preservation of these herbs. If they don't give you specific ways that they practice sustainability such as mentioning the farms that they purchase from, don't buy from them. Corporations are the biggest reason for overharvesting of our natural resources. Let's take American ginseng (*Panax quinquefolius*) for instance. There are many states with rules for harvesting this herb, but there are people stealing ginseng from

private land and government land alike for the sole purpose of a quick buck. This is harming future availability of this herb. Not only that, but the companies that don't follow sustainability practices are also contributing to the demise of this herb for future generations. Sustainable companies will only buy American ginseng from farmers who grow that herb and not individuals harvesting from the wild.

4. **Only make medicine from sustainable resources or practices.** If an herb is on the at-risk list, it is considered best practice to either avoid using it or find alternative herbs with similar medicinal actions. You can either grow this herb yourself or purchase the herb from companies following sustainable practices. This guideline also includes harvesting at-risk herbs in a more sustainable way. If the root is popular or traditionally used to make medicine, see if the leaves/flowers/aerial parts could be used instead. A good example of this is with ghost pipe (*Monotropa uniflora*). The root is normally used (which will kill the plant), but herbalists have found that harvesting the aerial parts (following harvesting rules) will give you an identical medicine. This helps in the sustainability of this herb.

5. **Choose whole plant herbal preparations instead of essential oils.** This was discussed earlier and is important to herbalists, especially with at-risk plants. Frankincense (*Boswellia* spp.) is an at-risk herb that will be extinct if overharvesting continues at this rate. The resin itself can be used in less amounts rather than using the essential oil, or you can choose another herb that works similarly. Since large amounts of frankincense resin are needed to make an essential oil, this makes sustainability an issue to consider. Considering this example: why would you want to use large amounts of a plant when you can easily use a smaller portion to get the same benefit? You can get the same medicinal benefits from most plants in herbal preparations. It is appropriate to use essential oils as aromatherapy or add them to your ointments for aromatherapy and extra medicinal benefits, but not for all of your medicinal needs. I rarely use essential oils but have some in my cabinet to use on occasion.

If we all follow the harvesting rules and sustainability practices mentioned here, we will do our part in ensuring these plants are here for future generations. Keep these practices in mind as you develop your own apothecary and design your own herb gardens.

Exercise

Visit United Plant Savers online or talk to your local conservationist to find out which plants are at-risk or have a very small population in your area. Which plants are considered invasive where you live? Research each invasive plant and find uses for them as food or as medicine.

How many of the plants in your area are at-risk or endangered?

Chapter Eight
Harvesting from Herbs

There are multiple things to consider before harvesting from your plant. Is this the right time of year to harvest the part I need? Is it the right time of day to harvest? What parts do I need harvested? When is the plant available for harvesting? All of these questions involve some knowledge of each individual herb and will determine your harvesting schedule.

Mary's Advice
Before you begin harvesting, make sure you have the correct tools and that they are cleaned and sharpened after each use.

I keep a list of plants for each season that I need to harvest from and a separate list of medicines that need replenishing in my apothecary. Those herbs growing in abundance near me (or that I have grown myself) are put on the list to harvest. Those that are not in abundance, not growing in my area, or I can't grow myself are purchased separately from sustainable companies. I reevaluate this list yearly to determine if I can plant any herbs myself next year to reduce the need for purchasing. The more you do this, the more you will know how much of an herb is needed yearly for your use and whether or not you have the ability to grow or harvest that herb in your area.

A variety of tools make harvesting and collecting herbs easier, quicker, and more convenient. Each herbalist can decide on the price, quality, construction, and need for each of these tools. Some of the following tools are required while others are considered luxury or for convenience:

1. **Gloves**: I have different gloves for different needs in my home and business. I like rose gloves to harvest rose or raspberry/blackberry bushes. Your arms will thank you. However, using rose gloves makes it hard to

harvest petals or fruit because these gloves are thicker so it's harder to grab on to smaller parts of the plant. I have a pair of leather gloves when I am handling sharp or rough objects such as bark. I like vinyl gloves when I am harvesting in moist areas or rinsing roots, and regular cloth gloves when harvesting or handling other types and parts of plants. You will find your favorite kind to use as you gain more experience.

2. **Digging tools**: I have different sizes and types of digging tools for harvesting.

   a. **Pointed shovel**: I use this to help roots break through compacted dirt or to lift a whole plant with fibrous roots.

   b. **Trench spade**: I like this tool for digging taproots. You can dig deeper before the root breaks.

   c. **Digging/spading fork**: This tool is beneficial for loosening soil around branching roots and lifting them up without doing too much damage to the roots.

3. **Cutting tools**: There are many kinds of cutting tools. Each one is chosen due to the size of the leaf, flower, stem, or root being cut.

   a. **Basic pruners**: These come in different sizes and are my first choice to harvest leaves, flowers, or aerial parts of herbs. I have a couple of different sizes.

   b. **Snippers**: These are similar to scissors but are smaller to handle and usually come with a case to protect the blade and possibly a locking mechanism. I use these to harvest smaller kitchen herbs.

   c. **Loppers**: These are larger pruners for larger and thicker branches. I use these to cut downed trees or shrub branches.

   d. **Pruning saw**: I rarely need to use this, but it does come in handy when it is time to prune a tree or shrub and also when a branch breaks and it needs help coming down.

   e. **Knives**: I use both a pocketknife and a weeding knife. The pocketknife is handy for cutting slits on tree branches, and the weeding knife is very handy to cut through some roots to harvest another root you want. It can also help in removing some stones or rocks around the root. Another knife I use is a standard kitchen knife for chopping. I use this to chop up my roots into smaller pieces.

4. **Containers**: You will need some kind of container or bag to carry your harvest back home. Some people will use one container to harvest

different herbs, and some people prefer to have different containers for each. You could also carry some mason jars to fill right away with your harvest to make herbal preparations immediately when you get back.

5. **Bristled brush**: I use an old toothbrush, or you can use a vegetable brush to clean off roots.

6. **Miscellaneous items**: These could be added for convenience or for comfort and include kneepads, gardening carts or wagons, gardening stools, gardening belts, aprons, or backpacks.

Mary's Advice

When you are first learning when to harvest the different parts of an herb, shrub, or tree, begin by making a chart (an Excel sheet or a journal works well). Include the plant parts along the top, and the months to harvest down the side, then fill this chart with the herbs and their parts that you wish to make medicine with. This chart acts as a reference during the year for what you need to be harvesting each month.

Now that we have talked about the kinds of tools needed for harvesting, let's talk about the harvest itself. There are best times to harvest, best times to harvest certain parts of the plant, and best ways to harvest the plant. I will break down the harvesting process into plant parts:

1. **Leaves**: These are best collected in the morning once the dew has dissipated and before flowering. You will get optimal potency by collecting before the noon sun and before the plant puts its energy into the flowers and reproduction. There might be some plants that require you to collect the leaves as a young plant before they reach a certain height or maturity. An example would be stinging nettle (*Urtica dioica*), which needs to have its leaves harvested before it reaches a foot tall. This is usually in the spring. Dandelion (*Taraxacum officinale*) leaves are best collected as young leaves for food, but more mature leaves are preferred for medicine. To harvest leaves, either snip the petiole or snap it off if it comes off easily without breaking the stem.

2. **Flowers**: It is also best to harvest flowers in the morning after the dew dissipates and once the flowers first open for optimal potency. Some

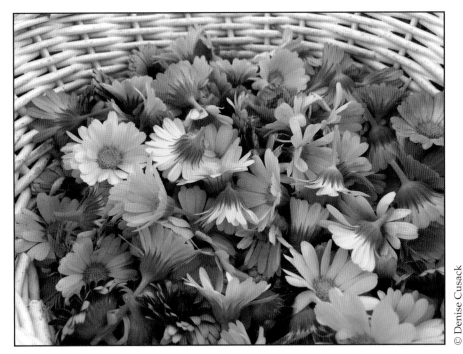

Calendula flowers

flowers continue to bloom throughout the year while others only bloom once. This is where knowing the blooming period is beneficial. Saint-John's-wort (*Hypericum perforatum*) is best collected when it first blooms on June 22nd or 23rd every year. The top four inches of the herb can be harvested, including the flowers, at this time. Calendula (*Calendula officinalis*) and chamomile (*Matricaria chamomilla*) both possess flowers that are utilized in herbalism. To harvest flowers only, cut just below the base of the flower, snap, or pull it off depending on the ease of removal.

3. **Roots**: The best time to dig roots is in the fall when the plant has set seeds and the energy has returned to storing food in the roots. Late afternoon is the preferred time to harvest roots since the energy has returned to the soil at that time. To harvest roots, make sure that there are plenty of other plants in the vicinity, you have collected and scattered seeds, and try to dig deep enough to go under the roots.

4. **Aerial parts or "herb"**: Some herbs can be harvested by their aerial parts. When you are researching a particular plant and it is mentioned

that the part to be used medicinally is the herb, this means that you can harvest the flowers, leaves, and stem. To harvest the aerial parts, cut no more than ⅓ of the plant just above a set of leaves at an angle. Whichever side of the angle is higher, the axillary buds will grow a new shoot in that direction. I usually cut the stem with only two or three sets of leaves on it when harvesting, depending on how tall the plant is. Collect Saint-John's-wort aerial parts and dry them on a screen out of direct sunlight in mid-June.

🌿 If you can, add this herb to your apothecary now for remedies that will be made later in this book!

When you are beginning to harvest an herbaceous plant, it is good to know what kind of herbaceous plant it is. Is it considered an annual, biennial, or perennial? Perennials and annuals can be harvested according to the times listed above, but biennials have a different set of rules. Leaves of biennials are collected in their first year of growth. Roots of biennials are harvested at the end of the first year, and the flowers are collected in the second year. Do not try to harvest biennial roots in the second year because they are mushy or dead at that point.

When harvesting annuals, only cut back to four inches so they will grow back. This is important if you are wanting more flowers. Perennials should only have ⅓ growth cut, and it is good to keep cutting the flowers to stimulate more production. Cutting the aerial parts by ⅓ will also produce more growth from the sides of the stem. This could help in leaf production too. Stop doing this by late summer so the last flowers produced will produce seeds and multiply. To keep them from spreading/multiplying, cut the flowers.

Exercise

Make a list of the tools you already have and the ones you need in order to harvest herbs. Start collecting what you can for later use in this book.

Chapter Nine
Harvesting from Trees and Shrubs

There are many parts from a tree or shrub that we can harvest such as the leaves, flowers, bark, nuts, fruit, hulls, sap, resin, and roots. As with herbaceous plants, there are best times and seasons to harvest each along with best practices. Again, following harvesting rules should be uppermost in your mind, but there are a few more for this category. The first being you should never cut around the trunk (called girdling) to harvest bark because it will kill the tree. Second, it is best to harvest from recently downed trees or branches if possible. Each part of the tree and shrub are harvested differently and at different times.

1. **Leaves**: The best time to harvest leaves of a tree or shrub is after the dew dissipates and before flowering or with newly opened flowers if you are combining parts in your medicine. This timing follows the same as herbaceous plants. I like to make medicine with both the flower and the leaves with hawthorn (*Crataegus* spp.), so I will wait until the flowers open to harvest both. Some trees are mature and too tall for me to harvest from, so I will harvest leaves from saplings nearby. I could also wait until after a storm and check the area for downed branches. You can harvest the leaves by either breaking them off at the stem or cutting the petiole to the branch or woody stem. In the case of evergreens, you can cut them to the main branch or trunk (as in pruning) or pick them up after a storm.

2. **Flowers**: As with herbaceous plants, it is best to harvest flowers after the dew has dissipated and when they first unfurl and open. They are harvested by cutting the flowers directly from the branch or cutting just below the base of the flower.

3. **Fruit or berries**: Fruit or berries are the enlarged ovaries of the flowers that contain the seed(s). The timing of harvesting is different depending on the species. Some berries can be harvested in the summer, and some later in the fall. Make sure you research the herb to know the best time to collect the berries or fruit for consumption or medicine, and also know 100 percent of the identification before harvesting. You can usually just twist or pop off the fruit or berries when harvesting, but you can also cut them if needed.

4. **Bark**: The best time to harvest bark is either in the spring or fall when the sap is running to the branches or back to the roots. As stated above, you never want to harvest the trunk of a tree by cutting around it. You don't usually harvest from the trunk in most cases, but rather take from younger branches. It is very convenient for Mother Nature to help us out and leave it at our feet, and that is the absolute best scenario for collection. Cut a branch vertically lengthwise and make another vertical cut running parallel to the first cut to form a strip to peel. Cut horizontally on both ends of the vertical cuts and dig under with your knife until the section lifts at one end. You can then start peeling the strip from the branch. If smaller branches get in the way, you can cut them off. The inner bark can be peeled away from the

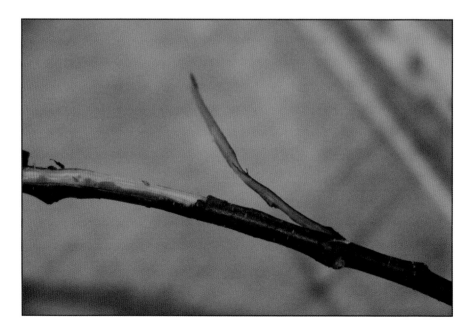

outer bark if required. Research the plant to see if the best part for medicine is the inner bark or the inner and outer bark combined.

5. **Nuts and hulls**: The best time to harvest nuts is late summer to early fall. Nuts are best collected as soon as they fall from the tree. Hulls (the fleshy part surrounding the nut) can be collected before they fall.

6. **Sap or resin**: Sap is collected in the spring to make syrup. It is thinner than resin. Resin is collected when the trunk or branch is damaged. You can see it ooze out to protect the tree. You can collect it by itself, or in the case of pine (*Pinus* spp.), you can also collect smaller branches containing the sap to make medicine.

7. **Roots**: I never harvest the roots of a tree, especially if there are other parts of the tree with medicinal value. An exception would be sassafras (*Sassafras albidum*) root. Sassafras saplings are connected by their branching roots, which is why they are usually found in small groves. To harvest the root, you will need to loosen the soil near the top and find the connecting root. Once it is found, cut both sides of the connecting root far away from the trunk with a weeding knife and harvest the middle root. Neither sapling should be harmed doing it this way.

Keep in mind that medicine can be made out of different parts of trees and shrubs. Research your plant thoroughly to find the medicinal properties of each. Similar actions can be found in different plant parts but can vary in potency. Different parts can also affect the body in other ways, which is why researching a plant is so important before harvesting.

Exercise

Pick a tree in your area. Research the parts used to make medicine, the uses and medicinal actions of each part, and the best times to harvest those parts. Do this for other trees and shrubs around you and refer back to this information when making your own medicine in the future.

Chapter Ten
Fresh or Dried?

Are plants better used fresh or dried when making herbal preparations? Most people are under the assumption that fresh is always best or that dried is weaker, but that is not always correct. Sometimes, the plant is too strong taken fresh and needs to be dried for a milder action. Some herbs are best fresh, some are best dried, and others can be used either way. In the herbal community, you might hear how one herb is best when used fresh, but the dried plant material is just as good. The best course of action is to understand and know the herb you are using medicinally first. Research and experiment using that herb in different herbal preparations and come to your own conclusion.

Three good examples are lemon balm (*Melissa officinalis*), skullcap (*Scutellaria lateriflora*), and cascara sagrada (*Rhamnus purshiana*):

Lemon balm: This is an herb that we are taught to use fresh because the volatile oils are lost in the process of drying. The volatile oils have antimicrobial, nervine, and sedative properties. However, there is more to lemon balm than their volatile oils, and other constituents also have antimicrobial, nervine, and sedative properties. In *Gerard's Herbal*, John Gerard calls it "balme" or "bawme" and never mentions the use of fresh or dried leaves. He does talk about the smell being good for women who have the "strangling of the mother" (which I understand is anxiety with difficulty swallowing). He also says that "bawme" drunk in wine is good against the bitings of venomous beasts, comforts the heart, and drives away all melancholy and sadness.[7] We know today that the aromatic smell of lemon balm is due to the volatile oils, but he never mentions whether to use fresh or dried leaves in the wine.

In the *National Standard Dispensatory* from 1905, the authors never mention the use of fresh or dried leaves. They mention that the fragrance is lost after drying, but only consider the plant to contain ⅛ to ¼ volatile oil content.[8] In *The Complete Herbalist*, Dr. Brown states that boiling water extracts its virtues, but doesn't mention whether to use fresh or dried.[9] Neither of these authors mention the use of lemon balm as a nervine or sedative specifically either. What both of them do mention is that lemon balm is good for fevers. What we can take from this is that lemon balm has more than one property, more than one use, more constituents than volatile oils, and possibly more than one constituent responsible for antimicrobial and nervine qualities.

My experience has also proven to me that this herb is still effective as a nervine/sedative using dried leaves in herbal preparations. I have seen this effect in both water and alcohol extracts. Of course, lemon balm shouldn't be reduced to just a nervine/sedative herb. It has many other properties and uses. Interestingly, a study using the dried leaves (dried at room temperature) in an alcoholic base to determine activity on cancer cells found that they had an effect on cytotoxic and antiproliferative properties.[10] This means dried leaves had an effect on the death and spreading of these cancer cells. So, you do not have to use just the fresh leaves and stems of this herb, and it is not necessarily more potent or best to do so to get medicinal benefits.

Skullcap: Many people believe that skullcap is best used fresh, but this is more of a preference rather than necessity. It can be extracted in both water and alcohol and used either fresh or dried. According to Richo Cech in *Making Plant Medicine*, the parts used are "Entire aerial portions of the plant, including stems, leaves, and flowers, used fresh or dried." The fresh plant is preferred in a tincture, but the dried can be used. He continues to point out that both alcohol and water extracts can be used with either.[11] When I first started making herbal medicine and learning herbalism, I always used the dried leaves and noticed a relaxing effect. Then, I heard how it was best used fresh and decided to try and grow some myself. I made the tincture from fresh leaves and did not notice a huge difference except for the taste. I cannot say that it had a stronger relaxing effect than the dried leaves. What you can take from this is that people have their own preferences for herbal medicine practices. Do your diligent research and use both fresh and dried herbs in your herbal extracts if both are safe to be used. You will discover your own preferences in time.

Cascara sagrada: This herb should be dried before use and never used fresh due to the purgative effects it has on the body. Both lemon balm and skullcap are usually "best used fresh" but cascara sagrada is "never used fresh." This is a clear indicator of how to proceed when making medicine. If you research an herb and it states the parts used can be either fresh or dried, you can proceed to experiment with both. If in your research everyone tells you to avoid fresh parts or never use fresh, you should follow that procedure when making plant medicine.

Mary's Advice

When researching an herb, always start with older literature and materia medica for traditional uses and compare with the modern use of that herb, then look into any scientific studies about it. In the end, it will be your personal experience using an herb that solidifies your knowledge.

The common question as to whether fresh or dried is best is answered by considering the history of the herb in traditional medicine and how it is employed in modern herbalism today along with your own personal experience.

PART THREE
Plant Medicine

Chapter Eleven
Medicinal Properties of Herbs

In this chapter, you will learn about the medicinal properties of herbs and how they contribute to healing. Medicinal properties and medicinal actions are terms used interchangeably to describe an herb's actions in the body, and they can be used as adjectives to describe herbs as well. As you learn about herbs, you will discover more than one medicinal property associated with each. You will find that an herb can be strong in one action and weaker in another. They can have primary and secondary actions. You will also find that each property could be dependent on the type of herbal preparation you make or how each is extracted. Take your time to know and understand the following medicinal properties before moving forward in this book.

Mary's Advice
Get some index cards and write the name of a medicinal property on the front of each with the description of its action on the back. Use these flash cards to study.

The Properties
Adaptogen: It supports the body's immune system while helping the body deal with stress and its many effects.

Alterative: It corrects impure conditions of the blood by helping to support elimination channels of the body. Traditionally called "blood purifiers," alterative herbs work on a specific organ, system, or combination of areas in the body. They could also work on the liver, kidneys, lymphatic system, lungs, skin, or bowels by stimulating fluid activity or removing excess mucus. If you ask a group of herbalists for this definition, you might find different answers, but they all result in the same benefit and action. They restore function and vitality to the body by helping the body function properly.

Amphoteric: It balances function in the body. An amphoteric herb can help either high or low blood pressure or stimulate or lower the immune response. We sometimes call this modulating.

Analgesic: It alleviates pain when taken orally. Herbs work on different pathways to alleviate pain whether it is to relieve spasms, inflammation, relax nerves, etc. They do not always block pain receptors or prevent cells from producing prostaglandins the way pharmaceutical analgesics do.

Anodyne: Herbs with this property also alleviate pain but are used externally.

Anthelmintic: You will find many of these herbs with this property in parasite cleanse formulas. These herbs act against worms. There are other properties of herbs within this category that have specific actions on worms. A **vermicide** kills worms while a **vermifuge** helps in the expulsion of worms. In a good parasite formula, it will include both types of herbs. A **taenicide** kills a tapeworm and a **taeniafuge** causes the expulsion of the tapeworm. All anthelmintics are potent herbs and should be respected in their use.

Antifungal: The prevention or elimination of fungus.

Antilithic: Prevents the formation of urinary calculi (stones) and helps in their removal.

Antimicrobial: This medicinal property helps to resist, deter, or kill microorganisms. Most people use the terms antiviral, antibacterial, or antifungal to describe which specific microorganism an antimicrobial herb works on. These herbs do not always kill the organisms outright. They could work on the body's defenses (immune system) instead.

Antioxidant: Prevents oxidative stress or damage from oxidation.

Antiphlogistic: This property refers to the prevention or reduction of inflammation (in other words, **anti-inflammatory**).

Antiseptic: An herb that will help to prevent or counteract infection or the decaying of cells.

Antispasmodic: This means that the herbs will relax contracted muscular tissue (or spasms).

Anxiolytic: This term is used to describe an action to reduce anxiety.

Aperient: This property has a mild laxative action without the usual griping pain and stimulates the appetite and digestion. I feel comfortable using this category of herbs in smaller doses for children and the elderly.

Aphrodisiac: This term refers to increasing libido.

Aromatic: These are herbs with a strong fragrance or taste that tend to support the digestive, respiratory, and nervous systems. All aromatic herbs contain resins or volatile oils in their composition.

Astringent: This property tightens tissue when it is relaxed, weak, or injured. Herbs with this property will tighten and close a wound to stop the bleeding externally and restore structure to weak organs internally.

Bitters: This is a taste that refers to an action in the body, but herbalists use it to describe a property as well. This category stimulates digestive secretions and the entire process of the digestive tract to function properly.

Carminative: This property helps to relieve and dispel flatulence in the gastrointestinal tract.

Cathartic: This property has a stronger laxative action than an aperient. It can cause irritation and griping and is best combined with an antispasmodic to counter this effect. An herb can be both an aperient and cathartic based on the dose. Smaller doses will give an aperient action on the body, whereas a larger dose would offer a cathartic action. Larger doses should not be used for a long period of time.

Cell proliferant: This describes the ability to repair cells in the body. Our body can heal itself, but herbs with this medicinal property can help that process along.

Cholagogue: The action of this property is similar to bitters but is more specific to the stimulation of bile production and release in the liver and gallbladder.

Demulcent: This property soothes irritation or inflammation internally.

Deobstruent: The ability to remove obstructions in the body that prevent the flow of fluid.

Depurant: This refers to a purifying or detoxifying action.

Diaphoretic: This will increase perspiration to release heat or toxins.

Digestive: This aids the digestive system.

Diuretic: This increases the secretion and flow of urine.

Emetic: This property induces vomiting.

Emmenagogue: This property can regulate or induce menstruation.

Emollient: They soothe externally or act as a conditioner to the skin.

Errhine: Increases nasal secretions from sinus cavities.

Expectorant: This property promotes the discharge of mucus from the lungs.

Febrifuge: Contributes to a reduction in fever.

Galactagogue: The production of milk is increased.

Hemagogue: A property promoting the flow of blood.

Hemostatic: It reduces bleeding or stops it altogether.

Hepatic: A property referring to the liver.

Hypertensive: It can raise blood pressure.

Hypotensive: It can lower blood pressure.

Lactifuge: It can reduce milk flow.

Lithotriptic: This will dissolve kidney or bladder stones.

Lymphatic: A property stimulating the lymphatic system.

Mucilaginous: Plants that contain mucilage (gel-like polysaccharide substance in plants).

Nephritic: A property in reference to the kidneys.

Nervine: This property supports the nervous system. These can be sub-categorized as relaxing, stimulating, or tonic.

Nootropic: This property improves cognitive function and memory.

Nutritive: Plants that are nourishing to the body.

Parturient: It can stimulate uterine contractions to hasten childbirth.

Pectoral: These are healing to the lungs.

Purgative: A property that causes a strong evacuation of bowels with griping pains.

Refrigerant: These cool the body and relieve thirst.

Relaxant: This property will relax tension in the body.

Rubefacient: This property stimulates capillary dilation and redness while using external applications.

Sedative: This property creates a tranquilizing effect.

Sialagogue: It promotes secretion and flow of saliva (bitters produce this action).

Stimulant: It increases bodily functions.

Stomachic: It stimulates and tonifies the stomach.

Tonic: A property that strengthens and increases tone.

Trophorestorative: This is considered to be rebuilding, restorative, and nourishing.

Vulnerary: The ability to promote healing of wounds.

There is more to learning about medicinal properties than just knowing the definition. You need to understand how they work on the body, recognize how they contribute to healing different conditions, and be able to pick out the medicinal action that is needed for the body based on a condition.

Let's take, for example, vulnerary. The definition says that it promotes healing of wounds. How? It could help promote healing by stopping the bleeding, closing the wound, promoting cell regeneration, or preventing infections. How do vulnerary herbs contribute to different conditions? Vulnerary herbs could soothe pain or itching from an injury, help to regenerate new connective tissue and repair injuries, keep the wound from becoming infected, draw out any infections while helping to close the wound and stop the bleeding, or reduce any swelling. What conditions call for a vulnerary herb? This could include cuts, wounds, swellings, infected wounds, bleeding, burns, broken bones, abscesses, bed sores, and more. The following exercise will help you to achieve this understanding better.

Exercise

For every medicinal property above, answer the following:

- *What action does this medicinal property have on the body?*
- *How does this medicinal property help different conditions?*
- *What conditions call for this medicinal property?*

Be sure to keep this list handy when you learn about individual herbs and what kind of medicinal properties they have. You will eventually recognize which of them are needed for different conditions.

Chapter Twelve
Tools of the Trade

Before we talk about the different herbal preparations in the next chapter, I want to go over some common tools and ingredients you should have on hand in your workspace or kitchen. Not all of these tools are necessary to make medicine, but they could make the job a little easier. I will let you know which ones are not necessary, but rather helpful, in the description following the name of the tool so that you can be prepared to move forward in this book. You might already have many of these on hand.

> ### Mary's Advice
> The best way to use this section is to start collecting the necessary tools in preparation of making medicine later in this book when you are able to. Check them off as you go. In the next chapter, I discuss the different types of herbal preparations that you would use these tools for. You might find these tools available online, in stores, at thrift shops, garage sales, or flea markets. I have collected my tools over the years at some surprising places.

Tools
- **Apple corer**: This is a good tool to have to core your apples, but it also doubles as a lozenge cutter.
- **Blender/food processor**: I don't often use the blender or food processor unless I have very lightweight herbs that need blending in the menstruum (liquid that extracts the medicine). They are nice to have on hand when needed, but not a necessity.
- **Capsule machine and empty capsules**: These are not a necessity for this book, but you may wish to have these on hand if you want to make your own capsules using powdered herbs. If you do, be sure to match the right capsules with the machine.
- **Cheesecloth**: I use cheesecloth all the time to strain my herbal preparations. This can be found in the sewing or canning section of various stores.

- **Coffee grinder**: This is definitely on my necessity list to chop up hard, dried root material. I also use this to lightly pulse herbs before I process them in herbal preparations.
- **Containers and bottles**: You will want an assortment of containers to hold your finished products and different sizes of bottles to store your extracts. The glass bottles and containers should be darker colored (blue or brown) for protection from light. Always store herbal preparations in a cool, dark area for extended shelf life and potency. Below is a list of basic containers and bottles you might need. You can order any specialty container or bottle that you wish to work with later.
  - Lip balm tubes
  - 4 ounce and 9 ounce glass containers
  - 1 ounce and 2 ounce glass bottles with droppers
  - 4 ounce glass bottle with atomizer (spray attachment)
  - 8 ounce and 16 ounce bottles with caps
- **Cotton balls**: These are always good to have on hand, especially if you are applying any oil in the ear, or for external application of oil preparations.
- **Cotton diapers**: I use these for external fomentations. However, you can use any white dish towel or other cloth material that you have on hand. I prefer mine with no coloring or bleach.
- **Cutting board**: A good wooden or glass cutting board is preferable to cut up herbs and protect the countertops.
- **Double boiler**: I utilize this tool to make infused oils and ointments/salves. Some people prefer to use slow cookers (which you can use instead). I don't personally use slow cookers because the heat setting doesn't go low enough for my preference. If you use one, you will want to monitor the oil so it doesn't burn.
- **Glass eyecups/shot glass**: You can purchase glass eyecups specially designed to fit around the eye or you can just use a shot glass (make sure you have a towel handy). With either one, they need to be sterilized between each use, and only use one per eye each time.
- **Foot bath basin**: This is not a necessary tool, but it is convenient. Foot baths sometimes offer massage options or heat up the water depending on the model. I was given one for a gift and utilize it to soak

my feet in herb-infused water. You can also use a bathtub or a large container.

- **Funnels**: I have a couple different sizes to add my herbal preparations into containers or bottles.
- **Glass bowls**: I prefer to use glass bowls to mix my herbs in, but you could use ceramic or stainless steel too.
- **Heating pad/hot water bottle**: It is sometimes beneficial to use a low-setting heating pad or an old-fashioned hot water bottle with external applications of herbal preparations.
- **Infusers, various sizes**: An infuser makes it simpler to remove herbs from water without straining. I have a larger one to make pots of infusions for the bathtub or fomentations, one that will sit in my teapot, and one for a mug/teacup.
- **Kitchen scale**: Make sure you have one that measures both grams and ounces.
- **Knives**: You could have a few different sizes, but I mainly use a large chopping knife specifically for herbs.
- **Labels**: This is a necessity for labeling different herbal preparations. I use standard address labels, but you can also get labels specific to your containers or bottles.
- **Mason jars**: I use pint, quart, and gallon mason jars depending on the need.
- **Measuring cups/spoons**: Keep a separate set of these for just your herbs (not for food).
- **Mortar and pestle set**: I have both a small and large set to crush my herbs.
- **Muslin bags**: A very convenient product for infusing herbs in a bathtub.
- **Plastic wrap**: This is useful to have for covering fomentations or jars containing apple cider vinegar.
- **Pots and pans, assorted sizes**: I use separate pans for herbal preparations in various sizes.
- **Roll gauze**: To have on hand when making poultices.
- **Rolling pin**: A small rolling pin is used to roll out herbal lozenges.
- **Rubber bands**: I use rubber bands to hold bunches of herbs together as I dry them.

- **Rubber gloves**: The only time I use these is when I am harvesting and making herbal preparations with black walnuts or other herbs that dye the skin.
- **Scissors**: Have these handy for cutting purposes.
- **Spoons (wooden or stainless steel)**: Have some to mix or stir herbs.
- **Strainers, various sizes**: I have a strainer to fit my bigger pot, one that fits a 4-quart measuring cup, and one that is smaller to strain a cup.
- **Suppository/bolus mold**: Not necessary unless you want to make your own herbal bolus or suppositories.
- **Tea bags**: Not necessary unless you wish for convenience.
- **Teacups**: Not necessary to drink tea, but definitely more pleasurable to drink tea or tisanes from. You can easily drink your herbal tea from a mug too.
- **Teakettle**: Another tool that isn't necessary, but I love one with a whistle. You can easily boil water in a pan or electric teakettle instead.
- **Teapot**: I like having a teapot to make more than one cup at a time.

Ingredients
- **Apple cider vinegar with the mother**: I use organic apple cider vinegar to make my medicine. This can be a good menstruum as an alternative to alcohol depending on the need.
- **Beeswax**: I prefer using the pastilles after learning the hard way. Cutting a block of beeswax is time consuming (not to mention hard on your hands), plus it takes longer to melt the larger chunks.
- **Cocoa butter**: I include this ingredient in my lip balm formula and lotions. It is best to get unrefined and organic cocoa butter. For ease of use, try purchasing wafers.
- **Cold-pressed extra-virgin olive oil, coconut oil, or other oils that you prefer**: I prefer to use organic in any oil that I use on the skin. I like to use olive oil for my ointments, but you can use any oil as a base. Do some research and choose the oil that fits your needs best.
- **Distilled water**: I like to use this type of water so it doesn't have any competing minerals or additives.
- **Essential oils (optional)**: I will add essential oils to my ointments or salves for aromatherapy or for additional actions. However, they are not necessary in herbalism.

- **Raw local honey**: Using unpasteurized local honey is best for medicinal uses. Try your best to get honey from a local beekeeper, orchard, or health food store. The grocery store should be the very last option, but it will do if you have no other resource.
- **Vegetable glycerin**: I like to purchase organic made from non-GMO soy.
- **Vodka (100 proof), grain alcohol (190 proof), and brandy (80 proof)**: I will use each one of these when needed in my herbal preparations as a menstruum or a preservative. Organic is best but purchase what is available to you.

Chapter Thirteen

Herbal Preparations

This chapter discusses the different forms of herbal medicine used in herbalism that are referred to as herbal preparations. Some of these preparations can be used as internal, external, or both internal/external applications. You will have a chance to make these herbal preparations throughout the exercises in this book. I will explain how each is used below.

- **Acetum**: This is an extract using vinegar. Vinegar is a good menstruum, but it doesn't have as long of a shelf life as alcohol or vegetable glycerin, and it doesn't extract all the constituents. It is often used as a replacement for alcohol and to extract nutrients and certain aromatic constituents. Make it similar to a tincture, but with vinegar instead of alcohol.
- **Bath**: An herbal bath requires a person to soak in an infusion of herbs and warm water to receive medicinal benefits. An herbal infusion can be prepared and poured directly into the bath, or a muslin bag holding herbs can be placed under the running water and steeped in the tub before use.
- **Bolus (or suppository)**: An herbal bolus is used when an herb needs to be inserted into an orifice of the body. Powdered herbs are added to melted coconut or cocoa butter and mixed to make a paste. They are then shaped into a bolus roughly an inch long and about the width of your little finger. There are convenient molds to help shape this herbal preparation as well. Boluses can be stored in the refrigerator or the freezer before use.
  Soothing antifungal/antimicrobial bolus:
  1. Melt ½ cup unrefined cocoa butter.
  2. Add powdered calendula flowers (page 108) to the melted cocoa butter and stir until it creates a paste that can be formed, or mix 2 tablespoons calendula-infused oil to the

melted cocoa butter and pour this into a bolus mold and skip the next step.
3. Shape into the length mentioned above.
4. Freeze until needed. This bolus can be soothing to vaginal yeast infections, help minimize excess candida, or heal tissue in the anal cavity.

🌿 Another remedy added to your apothecary!

- **Cold infusion**: This is an herb steeped in cold water for a length of time. A cold infusion could bring on different actions compared to a tisane (warm infusion), depending on the herb and the action needed. I like to add roughly 1 cup cold water with 1 ounce herb in a pint jar and steep overnight.
- **Concentrated preparation**: This is a stronger preparation that reduces the volume of an infusion or decoction. I was taught that if you simmer an infusion or decoction until you have ½ the volume you started with, it is considered "the third power." If you simmer your preparation until you have ¼ the original volume, it is considered "the seventh power." Infusions and decoctions are more potent this way. To preserve a concentrated preparation, add ¼ the volume with vegetable glycerin and refrigerate it.
- **Creams/lotions**: Some herbs can be infused into an oil and added into a cream or lotion, depending on the ingredients. Lotions are lighter in weight and have more water content than creams. Creams have a higher concentration of oil.
- **Decoction**: This herbal preparation is chosen when extracting thicker plant material like roots, dried berries, seeds, and bark. In a small pot, mix 1 ounce dried herbs or 2 ounces fresh herbs with 1 quart cold water and bring it to a low simmer. Simmer this for 20 minutes, take it off the heat, let it steep for another 20 minutes, then strain the liquid.
- **Douche**: This application uses an herbal infusion or decoction and is inserted into the vagina using a fountain syringe.
- **Electuaries**: This preparation consists of powdered herbs mixed with something sweet for palatability such as honey or vegetable glycerin. Electuaries can be taken by the spoonful or added to a warm beverage.
- **Elixir**: This is a sweetened alcohol extract. Honey can be added to the tincture when it is being prepared or once it is strained.

- **Enema**: This application uses an herbal infusion or decoction, and the liquid is dispersed into the anus.
- **Extract**: This term describes herbal preparations made with a liquid in order to extract constituents from herbs. The process of extraction is called maceration. The herb is called the marc, and the liquid is called the menstruum. The herbs soak in the liquid for a period of time and this is called macerating. An extract could be made using water, alcohol, vegetable glycerin, or apple cider vinegar.
- **Fomentation**: This is the process of dipping a natural cloth in a warm infusion or decoction and placing it externally on the affected part of the body for a period of time. Once it covers the affected part of the body, you can place plastic wrap over it to keep the moistened heat in longer and secure it with an Ace bandage. The moist heat gets the medicinal property of the herb to the area quickly. I often use these in overnight applications.
- **Glycerite**: This is an extract using vegetable glycerin as the menstruum. They are often used for children or those who wish to avoid alcohol. Vegetable glycerin has a sweet taste that children love. A good rule of thumb is to use 100 percent vegetable glycerin with fresh herbs and 60 percent vegetable glycerin with 40 percent water with dried herbs. Pack the jar when using fresh herbs, and only fill half the jar when using dried herbs since they will expand in time. Fill the jar with either vegetable glycerin or a mix of vegetable glycerin and water. Cap, label, and let it macerate for one month while shaking it daily.
- **Infused honey:** This herbal preparation uses raw honey and a little bit of heat to extract an herb.
- **Liniment**: An external use of an extract using alcohol, witch hazel, or vinegar.
- **Oil**: This refers to an herbal-infused oil used externally on the skin. Every oil has different benefits, according to your needs. There are two ways to make an oil and it can be quick or take 2 weeks. Fill a clean glass jar with ½ to ¾ dried herbs and fill the rest with the oil. Push any air out and cap tightly. Place this in the sun for two weeks and shake daily. A quicker way is to use a double boiler or slow cooker. For example, try chopping up 4 to 6 garlic (*Allium sativum*)

cloves, placing them in the top of a double boiler, and pouring in enough olive oil to cover the garlic. Add water to the bottom of the pan and simmer on low for about an hour or two. When that is finished, strain, cool, and place the garlic-infused oil in a bottled jar. Remember to always label your finished products.

🌿 You just made an important first aid herbal preparation for your apothecary!

Research the benefits of garlic used externally. The most important thing to remember when you are making infused oils is that water doesn't mix with oil! If fresh herbs are used like garlic, the water in them could grow bacteria. That is why I only make small amounts of garlic-infused oil at a time, and I make a new batch after a couple of months. There are some herbal oils that are considered best when using fresh herbs, but I have made them with dried material and they work just as well. If you do choose to use fresh herbs, wilt them for at least a day before infusing them in the oil. Fresh garlic is the only herb I do not wilt or dry before using.

- **Ointment/salve**: This is an herbal oil with added beeswax to help solidify it. Usually, 1 ounce beeswax is used with every 2 cups oil to make a soft ointment. Place water in the bottom of the pan with the oil in the top pan of a double boiler. Add the beeswax and simmer this until the beeswax is melted. I pour it immediately into a container and let it cool. Remember to always label your finished products.
- **Oxymel**: This is a vinegar extract with the addition of honey. Fill a mason jar with herbs, pour in organic apple cider to the top, and put on the jar lid (first placing a barrier such as plastic wrap or wax paper between the metal and apple cider vinegar). Label the jar and store it on the counter for a month, shaking daily, then strain. Once it is strained, honey can be added for taste (I recommend ¼ to ½ honey to the total volume of liquid in the jar).
- **Plaster**: An external application of powdered or dried plant material is moistened and placed onto a cloth and secured.
- **Poultice**: This is made with fresh herbs applied directly to the skin. Bruise the fresh herb by chewing or crushing it, then apply it to the skin. Secure it with gauze and/or an Ace bandage so it doesn't move.

- **Steam**: This process uses steam from an aromatic herbal infusion to deliver its medicine. A warm infusion is made using the aromatic plant, and the lid is removed while your face hovers over top of the infusion. A towel is used to keep the steam located around your head. Steams are recommended for respiratory congestion or mucosal tissue moistening and healing.
- **Succus (succi plural)**: Plant juices are used medicinally either internally or externally. It is often harvested by blending or mashing the plant and squeezing the juice through a cheesecloth or using a press. It is sometimes necessary to add a small amount of water when using a blender. This expressed juice can be preserved by adding a small amount of alcohol or vegetable glycerin.
- **Syrup:** This preparation adds honey to an infusion or decoction.
- **Tisane or warm infusion:** A warm water extract. This herbal preparation is mostly used with the softer portions of an herb such as leaves or flowers. It is often mistakenly referred to as "herbal tea," but the parts used are not from the plant species *Camellia sinensis* (tea plant). Tisane or warm infusion would be the correct term to use when using water to extract other herbs. Pour the boiling water over the herb, cover it, and let it steep for 15 to 20 minutes. Extraction times may vary. This preparation can be taken internally or used externally as a wash, fomentation, or bath.

Mary's Advice

Some herbalists prefer to work with tinctures because of their convenience and shelf life while others rely more on infusions and decoctions due to their traditional uses in herbal medicine. It is perfectly fine to work with all or just a few of these preparations, depending on the availability of ingredients or your ability to make them.

- **Tincture**: This is an extract using alcohol as the menstruum. The folk method doesn't measure first and instead uses fresh herbs packed to the top of a mason jar or dried herbs filled halfway to the top. I like to grind my herbs first. You can also add the herbs and alcohol into a blender before maceration. I use either 190 proof grain alcohol or 100 proof vodka, depending on the herb's constituents (research to find the proper amount of alcohol content for each herb). A menstruum chart can be used to determine how much alcohol content is needed for each extraction.

Alcohol content is determined by dividing the proof in half. So, 100 proof is automatically 50 percent alcohol content with 50 percent water content. All you need to do is fill the jar to the top with 100 proof vodka if 50 percent alcohol is needed. If fresh herbs are used, they sometimes need a higher alcohol content. I use grain alcohol and add water to balance it out. For example, if I need 75 percent alcohol for extraction, I will pour the 190 proof grain alcohol until it fills ¾ of the jar. I will fill the rest of the jar with water until it reaches the top.

Tinctures should be macerated in the jar for 4 weeks, give or take. This means you need to shake this extract once daily for four weeks. Afterward, strain the tincture through cheesecloth and squeeze out the excess. A press can be used when you are making larger amounts, or if you wish to get every bit of the tincture out of the herbs.

Chapter Fourteen
Doses and Measurements

The word "dose" refers to the measured amount of herbal medicine an individual consumes and how often it is taken. Dosage recommendations vary among herbalists based on their personal philosophies of distributing medicine. I like to use an assortment of philosophies in my practice and dose accordingly based on the herb and what I want to accomplish. Dosages could be higher in acute compared to chronic situations, for example, or a lower dosage could give a different action than a higher one. Oftentimes, I prefer to start at a lower dosage and move upward as needed. This is a great starting point for anyone learning herbalism until they better understand the actions of each herb on the body. Of course, the first thing you need to do before dosing with any herb is to research each one thoroughly. You will have a better understanding of the common dosages of herbs this way. We will discuss herbs more thoroughly in Part Five of this book.

> ## Standard Doses
> **Tinctures**: 30–60 drops, 3 times daily (or 5 times daily if needed)
> **Infusions/decoctions**: 1 cup, 3 times daily
> **Vinegars**: 1 tablespoon, up to 5 times daily
> **Glycerites**: Double the tincture standard dose
> **Syrups/Succi:** 1 tablespoon, up to 5 times daily

There are many different philosophies when it comes to dosing. Each philosophy differs in its approach to herbal medicine, and when you understand where each philosophy originates, you will come to understand that all of them can be properly utilized. I will explain how Western herbalism views dosing and the different philosophies that it follows.

The first philosophy believes that very small amounts of an herb can be beneficial and have fewer risks. This is called drop dosing when tinctures are used. A drop dose of 1 to 5 drops would be the starting point,

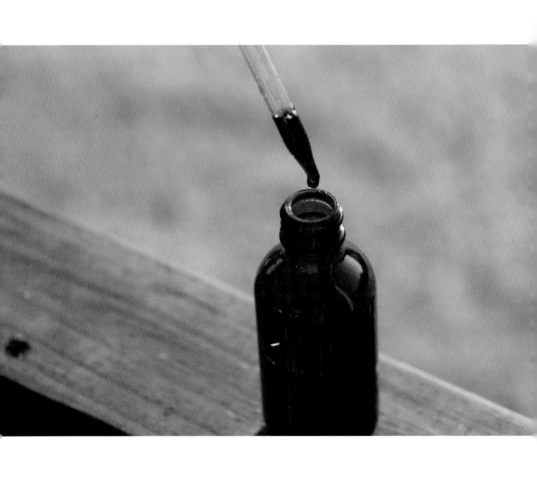

according to this philosophy. Using fewer than 10 drops is balancing to an individual on many levels, and anything more than 10 drops provides definitive medicinal actions on the body. Drop dosing is also used with what we call low-dose botanicals or herbs that should only be used by experienced herbalists and in minute amounts.

Another philosophy considers how powerful herbs can be and usually follows a standard dose of an herb. All standard doses are for adults weighing 150 pounds and can be adjusted according to the individual's weight. A child weighing 75 pounds would consume one half the standard dose. Many believe this is a good starting point, but I will often start with less and only increase the dose or frequency if needed. This dosing practice works well in chronic cases or in situations that need a gentler approach.

The third philosophy utilizes the absolute maximum dose that can be given. The tincture would be dosed at 100 drops (5 milliliters) instead of 30 drops, 3 times daily. This could bring a quicker result when needed in the case of acute situations.

Mary's Advice

Most of the time, you can use the standard dose of an herbal extract to begin with, unless the herb is considered low dose. This is why it is always better to research the herbs first.

I utilize all three of these philosophies since I see many types of situations and needs in individuals. If I believe there is an emotional need, such as a broken heart, I would utilize a drop dose of tincture or even a flower essence instead. I normally begin standard dosing of tinctures at 10 to 20 drops, 3 times daily and increase as needed, depending on the individual and the situation. A lot of times, the smaller dose is enough, especially for longer periods. If an individual is in a lot of pain, I will use the last philosophy and dose at the maximum level.

Dosages can vary with each type of herbal preparation, even when they are made using the same herb. The dose of a tincture, warm or cold infusion, vinegar, or glycerite will generally be different depending on the menstruum used. Tinctures are considered stronger medicine than infusions/syrups, glycerites, or vinegars/oxymels. Because of this, tinctures are dosed in smaller amounts. Tinctures and glycerites are often measured in drops, teaspoons, or milliliters. Vegetable glycerin is not as strong of a menstruum as alcohol, so doses of glycerites are commonly doubled compared to tinctures made with the same herb. Infusions are measured in cups, teaspoons, or ounces. Oxymels, syrups, and vinegars are measured in ounces, teaspoons, tablespoons, and sometimes even shot glasses! (Thank you, grannies everywhere.)

Common Equivalents in Dosing

20 drops = 1 milliliter
1 teaspoon = 5 milliliters
1-ounce dropperful = 20 drops
1-ounce bottle = 30 milliliters
2-ounce dropperful = 40 drops

There is yet another form of dosing called pulse dosing that integrates taking breaks in ingesting the herb. This can be useful for long-term use of an herbal preparation to either give the body a rest, let the body adjust on its own, or keep the body from relying on an herb for a particular action. Pulse dosing could include either avoiding the herb or formula altogether or replacing the herb with a different one for a period of time. Some herbs are not meant to be taken as a preventative or for long periods of time like pharmaceutical medicine does and should be removed periodically before resuming. I have done this when I believe a break is needed.

So far, we have mentioned how to dose the volume of herbs in liquid extracts. Oftentimes, you will see dosing in terms of weight when dry herbs or capsules are used. For example, you might read that 2 to 4 grams of a particular herb are recommended daily. That is easy to figure out if you are using only one herb, but it will take some math to figure out how much of each additional herb a formula contains in every dose.

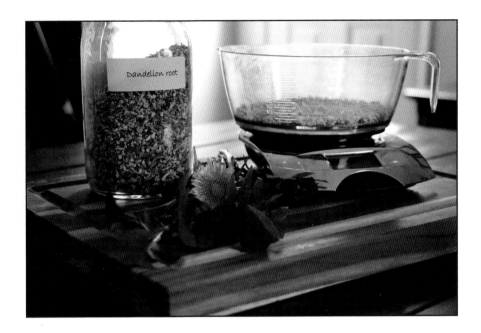

Herbs are measured in doses when distributing medicine, but measurements are also necessary to create consistency in herbal formulas or when instructing others on how to make different herbal preparations. Herbs are measured in ounces, grams, or parts. It is common instruction when making an infusion to mix 1 ounce herb with 1 cup water. However, 1 ounce is different with every herb or part used. If I am making a formula, I will weigh the individual herbs first or combine the parts and then place them in the infuser.

When combining herbs in a formula, a practitioner might call for the formula to include a number of parts consisting of each herb. The "part" could be any measurement you choose such as a cup or tablespoon. If the formula calls for 2 parts nettle leaves and 1 part rose petals, you could substitute the word "part" for "cup" instead. Therefore, the formula would be 2 cups nettle leaves and 1 cup rose petals. Obviously, various metrics could be used depending on your culture, how you are taught, or the country that you live in.

Mary's Advice
This book will focus on teaching the folk method to make the process of learning easier for beginners.

There are different techniques of measurement that herbalists use when making herbal preparations. Each of these techniques is based on how the herbalist was taught and whether or not the herbal preparations will be sold on the market. The folk method is a simple but very effective way of preparing herbal medicine where measuring isn't precise or even necessary. This method calls for eyeballing measurements and adjusting the dosages as needed for each individual. I follow this technique in my practice. The dosage might need to be adjusted to get the desired result, but it should work every time.

Another technique uses the same amount of herb to menstruum every time when making the product. This works well in commercial products if you are selling to the masses and want to make sure they are made exactly the same each time. I use this technique when I provide formulas that will be sold on the market. This might also be beneficial for the herbalist expecting the same results every time they make it. Similar doses, however, don't always work the same for every individual, and the same herb could have a different level of constituents in them from year to year. Even if you use the exact herb to liquid ratio, it is almost impossible to get the exact same constituents or potency extracted every time you make the herbal preparation. This could be due to environmental changes, different harvesting times, purchasing the herb from different places, harvesting the herb in a different place, etc.

The practice of weighing each herb or combination of herbs in any herb to menstruum ratio is only necessary in standardization processes or when you are making products for the mass market. Standardization is the guarantee that the medicine contains the same amounts of active constituents every time it is made. This process of making medicine is reserved for dried/raw plant material in products sold on the market. As I mentioned before, herbs cannot be guaranteed to contain the exact same amounts of constituents, but by using formulas, you can come close. The herbalist who is concerned with the potency of different constituents in the tincture will want to measure precisely to yield a consistent product batch after batch. The herbalist wanting to practice in a more traditional manner will use the folk method and know that no matter how it is prepared, the medicine will work. The difference is in the doses, and both techniques are considered correct ways to practice medicine making. It is more about your consistency of practice rather than the consistency of an herb.

Exercise

Choose an herb of your choice and research the standard dose and maximum dosages used along with the medicinal properties it has. Consider the three different philosophies outlined above. In what situations would you use the first, second, and third philosophies?

PART FOUR

Basic Understanding of Energetics in Herbalism

Chapter Fifteen
Why Energetics?

Energetics in herbalism is the use of descriptions of plants and people to determine the correct herbs for an individual. Patterns are observed and utilized in order to create homeostasis (maintaining stability in the body) between an individual and herbs. The energetics from the person and the plant are matched so that each can balance the other using opposite qualities. You balance heat with cold, or dry with moisture, for example, to maintain stability. Energetics are important to help balance the body. To me, the practice of energetics is a key component of herbalism and understanding this component is the difference between being an average herbalist and a great one.

Mary's Advice

I focus on the four qualities and tastes of an herb along with the tissue states and constitution of each individual for the purpose of teaching the understanding of energetics in this book, but I recommend you expand your learning about the history of energetics and energetic patterns from additional sources as well.

In almost all ancient traditional medical systems, energetics is considered when analyzing a plant and matching it to the need of an individual. You might have heard of yin-yang, the three doshas, the five elements, the four qualities, the tastes of herbs, or names of tissue states such as atrophy. All of these are energetic patterns that are used to help choose the right herb. In *Culpeper's Complete Herbal*, Nicholas Culpeper describes herbs by their "governments and virtues," which uses the ruling planets along with an herb's taste and qualities to explain their actions on the body. He used astrology to correlate different body parts to a planet.[12] Some herbalists still use this form of energetics, but I have never learned it myself.

Another form of energetics is the doctrine of signatures, which matches the herb to an organ of the body. This form of energetics does not balance the body by the use of opposing patterns, but rather matches the herb to the organ system that is in need of repair or strengthening. Using the doctrine of signatures requires the use of observation instead of memorizing or learning about an herb in a class. The herbalist will look at a plant and search for similarities between plant parts and body parts. An example would include Solomon's seal (*Polygonatum* spp.) root, where observation of the root itself resembles that of the disks in the spine. Therefore, the use of Solomon's seal benefits the spine using the doctrine of signatures. As a matter of fact, Solomon's seal is a cell proliferant that helps in the repair of connective tissue and is specifically indicated for disk injuries. I do not consistently rely on the doctrine of signatures for choosing an herb, but I do like to document them as I am journaling about a plant. It is fun for me to see what I come up with and compare it to medicinal properties of that herb. I once journaled about sweet leaf (*Monarda fistulosa*) and noticed how each of the petals along with the small hairs at the tips and base of the petals seem to reach in all directions. All I could think about was how our nerves

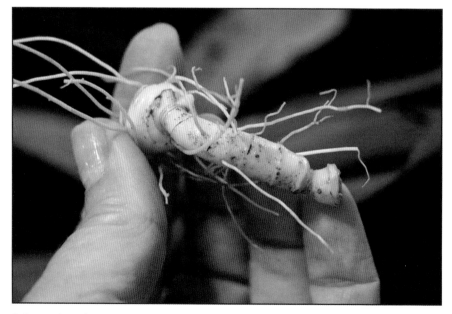

Solomon's seal root

connect and reach in all directions in our body. Sweet leaf is a powerful relaxing nervine.

Other forms of energetics are used today based on the culture, belief system, or educational training of the herbalist. The elements can be used to describe plants and people, and each can have certain qualities and connections to the four qualities, organs in the body, or four temperaments. Tastes are commonly used in both Eastern and Western herbalism for the understanding of how an herb will work in the body. Food can be a valuable tool for balancing individuals. Keep in mind that no particular diet is right for everyone, and choosing the best herb or food for an individual will be more effective than choosing an herb or food for a specific condition. Energetics are utilized in herbalism to choose the best herb that will be effective for the individual based on their own body's needs.

Chapter Sixteen
Plant Energetics

Plant energetics are comprised of both certain flavors or tastes and the qualities from each plant can produce an action within the body. This could also include planet or element associations and the doctrine of signatures. Each plant has a combination of tastes, or one distinct taste, that will give the indication of what the herb is best used for. Not only that, but each plant also has a certain quality associated with it based on the action it has, the constituents it contains, or how it feels within or upon the body. *Organoleptic* is a term that is used to describe what effect herbs have on the body by using the senses, or how the herb feels within the body by using taste, touch, sight, or smell. Medicinal properties were already listed in Chapter Eleven (page 49), and you will have a better understanding about the plant constituents as you study each one. Once you have experience working with individual plants, you will understand the tastes and qualities of each better. Here, I will describe what the tastes and qualities are, and how they are used in herbalism.

Plants have distinct tastes that can help to determine how they will act on the body. They include bitter, sweet, sour, salty, pungent/spicy, acrid, and bland. I have heard others describe astringent (drying) as another taste; however, I personally see that as a quality and a medicinal property. These tastes can give a good indication of what kind of medicinal action the herb will have within the body, and how the herb can balance the body's overall energetics. It is always good practice to know the correct identification of an herb if you are out wildcrafting, and you will want to know whether the plant is toxic or potentially poisonous first before you ever put it in your mouth. You know what they say about tasting mushrooms in the wild? All mushrooms are edible, but some only once! I am not sure where that saying came from, but I have heard it often. This could go for herbs as well in certain parts of the world where deadly plants are growing in the wild. In my area, you will come across water hemlock (*Cicuta douglasii*). This plant can be confused with many

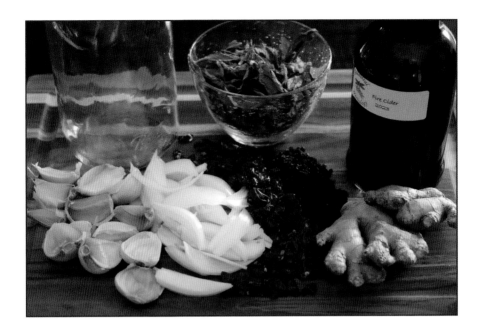

other similar looking plants. Be 100 percent sure of your identification before trying to taste them.

I personally love tasting herbs and adding them to my homemade meals for medicinal and culinary needs or using the knowledge of taste to create the perfect tasting formula. As you gain experience with each herb, you will have more knowledge at your disposal. This becomes an adventure in itself, and it is fun experimenting with taste in your herbal blends. For example, you could play around with different ingredients that can contribute to different tastes and medicinal benefits in your fire cider. The exercise at the end of this chapter will help you to create your own fire cider, and you can repeat this exercise to create different versions of it. You can eventually decide which one you and your family like the best. Let's talk about these tastes and describe how they are used medicinally.

Mary's Advice

In order to understand the different tastes, experiment with food and herbs and document how they taste in a journal. You can guess what the herb or food does medicinally and then double-check elsewhere to see if you are correct. This will be a good reference for you as you continue learning herbalism and help enforce your capabilities as an herbalist.

Tastes

Bitter

You will sometimes hear the word bitters mentioned, which is a noun instead of an adjective. This noun refers to bitter tasting herbs being added to a liquid, oftentimes an alcoholic beverage or tincture, and taken prior to eating. In this case, the noun is the product of using a bitter tasting herb. The adjective is used to describe the taste itself. The bitter taste is usually referred to as unpalatable, disagreeable, or harsh; however, I disagree. I find that it is a distinct flavor that can become quite agreeable and palatable the more you taste it. It is an important taste that stimulates the digestion process, can increase appetite, and help with elimination. These bitter herbs are considered digestives because of this. Many of the bitter herbs also act as an anti-inflammatory, alterative, hepatic, sialagogue, cholagogue, and febrifuge. They are considered to be cooling to the body along with drying, but not always.

When I taste a bitter herb, I immediately think of the entire digestive tract benefiting from it. When the bitter receptors on the tongue are initiated, saliva is immediately increased. This is the first action in the digestive system preparing your body to get ready to eat and begin the digestion process. This is why bitter tasting herbs are considered as appetite stimulants. The body wants to take in nourishment once the tongue tastes something bitter. Other digestive secretions are increased including bile production and hydrochloric acid, the liver is stimulated and supported, and eventually the elimination channels are moved. With all of this in mind, bitter tasting herbs help with constipation, heartburn, flatulence, stomach pains, removing waste and toxins, bloating, low hydrochloric acid in the stomach, fevers, systemic inflammation, and much more. The notion in America that we should cover up bad tastes with something sweet and salty is actually doing a huge disservice to many that are living here. If you need the digestive action from a bitter tasting herb, do not cover up the taste with something sweet; otherwise, you will not get that action from the herb.

Sweet

This does not include processed sugar-laden treats in the diet. This is a taste found from naturally harvested food and herbs and is not comparable in taste to sugar. It can be a subtle sweetness coming from carrots, for example. I like to say that it is a pleasant flavor that makes you come back for more. Metaphorically speaking, maybe this is the herb's way of making sure the body continues to take what is much needed: nourishment.

Sweet herbs are tonics, trophorestoratives, and nutritives. They are often moist and cooling, and are considered demulcent and anti-inflammatory. They build and strengthen the body by providing much-needed vitamins and minerals for nourishment. Many are considered blood builders because of this. Vitamins and minerals are utilized to make energy in the body; therefore, these sweet tasting herbs are energizing. Many of our adaptogen herbs are considered sweet. Have you ever chewed a fresh red clover (*Trifolium pratense*) blossom? They are delicious added to a salad, and you should try one in order to get an idea of what sweet herbs taste like.

I will often use sweet herbs in a formula to balance out the harsh flavored herbs and make it more palatable. I am careful not to cover up all of the bitter taste if I need digestive or hepatic properties from the formula, and I will let clients know not to cover it up either. This is something to keep in mind as you are making your own herbal blends. Also, keep in mind that the individual can always add a little honey if they are disagreeable to the taste altogether and do not need the bitter action.

Sour

If you have ever sucked on a lemon, you will know this taste. Of course, in the world of herbs, this taste can often be less dramatic. Other words could be used to describe sour, such as tart or tangy. A tart cherry would be considered as having a sour taste. You will also find that the sour taste is not always thought of first. In the case of strawberries, we think they are sweet, but only once they are completely ripe. The taste of an herb can change with age, or with the herbal preparation. For example, dandelion leaves are often sweeter tasting when they are younger, and more bitter once they are older. The bitter taste can be brought forth in an infusion more with longer steeping time, which can happen with chamomile.

As you taste different herbs, you will also find that they can have multiple tastes. A lot of times, the sour taste is accompanied by sweetness, especially in fruits. The sour taste is derived from the acids contained in the herb such as tannic, citric, oxalic, or even ascorbic. The sour taste can also be noted in fermented foods and vinegars.

I consider sour herbs to be astringent, cleansing, and stimulating. They tend to tighten and strengthen tissue and prevent fluid from leaking both internally and externally. With this information, they are usually drying in nature and cooling. They can also have a stimulating or tonic effect on the liver or digestion. This can ultimately offer a cleansing action on the body. Anger is usually associated with the liver, and I do find it interesting that someone with a "sour disposition" is synonymous with being ill-tempered. Therefore, metaphorically speaking, sour tasting herbs could benefit individuals that are ill-tempered and full of rage.

Salty

This is a taste that many are familiar with, and some people even crave. The salty taste in herbs indicates that they have a high mineral content. Herbs with this taste generally act on the digestive tract and the kidneys. They can also have the ability to soften masses and help with elimination, which can be beneficial in cases of constipation. They can also stimulate the appetite, and in some cases, moisten and repair the tissue of the digestive system. They are usually considered cooling and moistening. Many of these herbs can also be drying in excess since most of them can be considered diuretics. The herbalist should know the individual herb well along with the taste each one has in order to understand this distinction.

Salty herbs can be considered diuretics, nutritives, and alteratives. They have been traditionally called "blood builders" or "blood purifiers." I find these herbs to be a necessary component in most of my formulas due to the impact they have on the process of elimination in the body, and how they add nutrition while helping to restore the functionality of the digestive system. I have found that this aspect is needed in many of my client's cases.

Some people think if we crave salt, it means that we are deficient in nutrients because these herbs are so substantial in minerals. This isn't necessarily the case. Some people just like the taste of salt the way someone craves sugar in our society. Sometimes, it is a way to combat stress or just have something to do (the need to munch, for example). Other times, it can be an indicator that there is an insufficiency in the adrenal glands (too much stress for long periods of time). Whatever the reason, remember moderation is best when it comes to this taste whether for sustenance or medicine.

Pungent

The words spicy and hot have often been used synonymously with this taste. However, not all pungent tasting herbs are considered spicy or hot. Pungency refers to a sharp and strong taste, and this can include many of our aromatic herbs that are frequently used in cooking. Have you tasted cayenne (*Capsicum* spp.), garlic, or rosemary before? All three have a sharp, pungent taste; however, only the cayenne is considered spicy and hot in cooking.

Mary's Advice

You want to also notice how an herb flows in your body. When you drink or taste and herb, sit back and feel if it moves up, out, in, or down throughout the body. This can help in knowing how an herb disperses itself, and what parts of the body are affected first. This information can be added to your journal.

Herbs with a pungent taste are very powerful movers and stimulants of the circulatory and digestive system. Each of these herbs have a warming effect on the body that increases fluid movement and can have a drying effect on tissue. They also help to increase activity in the brain, reduce muscle cramping, and help with bloating and flatulence.

Pungent tasting herbs are considered stimulants, diaphoretics, digestives, nervines, antispasmodics, and carminatives. I have mentioned previously that nervines support the nervous system, and they can be considered either stimulating or relaxing. Pungent herbs are usually considered stimulating nervines; however, some of the aromatic herbs can be considered relaxing nervines. Rosemary leaves can stimulate brain activity as a pungent herb and reduce anxiety. Sweet leaf (*Monarda fistulosa*) can stimulate digestion but can also be an ally to reduce tension and relax the nervous system. Pungent herbs such as cayenne and horseradish

(*Armoracia rusticana*) stimulate the senses, stimulate blood flow, and can stimulate the nervous system to increase energy and movement.

I like to add small amounts of pungent herbs to an herbal formula to help drive the medicine where it needs to go. I will also add them to balance the energetics of a formula when there is a need for a warming herb to balance the cold herbs.

Acrid

Acrid herbs create a biting and tingling sensation that will send shivers through your body upon first taste. It's not necessarily a taste as it is a sensation that is created from the herbs. They are usually considered low-dose herbs and can cause some mild to moderate nausea in larger doses. These acrid herbs tend to affect the nervous system to ease pain and tension and can offer antispasmodic properties.

Herbs such as lobelia (*Lobelia inflata*) and kava kava (*Piper methysticum*) fall into this category. Both of them are considered analgesic and relaxing nervines. A drop of either one of these tinctures will help you to identify this sensation. Acrid herbs are usually considered warming and drying to the body, but some could be considered cooling.

Bland

One would think that this isn't a taste at all, but a description of a lack of taste. That is a correct assumption. I will often see this with herbs abundant in mucilage. They are sometimes called neutral with moistening capabilities. The neutral means neither warming nor cooling to the body, and they tend to fall into the middle spectrum.

The Four Qualities

The four qualities can offer another way to understand the energetics of plants. They describe the way the plant feels in the body, and how this can contribute to balancing and healing of the individual. Each plant has two qualities out of the four—temperature and action. The temperatures are either warming or cooling, and the actions on the tissues are either drying or moistening. Both of these offer an inside look at how the herb can balance each individual's condition and overall constitution (more about this in the next chapter).

Upon first tasting an herb, the quality is almost instantaneous. You can feel if an herb is warming, cooling, drying, or moistening by how it feels on the tongue, how it feels when applied to the skin, or how it feels once it has been ingested. Have you ever had a burn and applied aloe vera (*Aloe vera* spp.) on it? How did it feel? I bet you would say cooling at first, and then moistening because it just feels moist. It certainly doesn't warm the burn further or dry it out. Therefore, aloe vera is a cooling and moistening herb. Since we described tastes, you could also taste aloe vera to find out that it tastes bland. These are the energetics of this particular plant. The intent of using these qualities is to balance the system. Care should be taken not to use these qualities in excess, or this can create an unbalanced condition. Moderation is the key.

> ### Mary's Advice
> Get that journal back out! Go back and taste the same herbs that you documented earlier. This time, instead of describing the taste or where the herb disperses in the body, document what two qualities out of the four each one has.

Warming Herbs

This quality of an herb tends to stimulate circulation and digestion while adding warmth to cold conditions or constitutions. These warming herbs usually affect the brain, the digestive tract, and the heart.

Warming herbs are used to balance cold conditions such as cold hands or feet, slow digestion, or loss of appetite. They can warm the system when there are chills, low energy, or any slow processes in the body. In excess, they can cause too much heat in the body in instances where they are taken for longer periods or in higher doses. This could also cause the body to dry out with so much heat.

Cooling Herbs

Cooling herbs are used to slow down processes in the body. They can reduce inflammation, counteract heat, and balance a warm constitution. They tend to affect the nervous system, stomach, and kidneys.

They are often utilized during fevers, hot flashes, arthritis, and other inflammatory conditions. They help to regulate heated conditions;

therefore, could reduce pain, reduce swelling, and strengthen tissue. In the nervous system, they will help in reducing anxiety, insomnia, or nervousness. All of these processes are in need of relaxing, reducing, or slowing down to prevent more damage from occurring. In excess, cooling herbs could slow down processes too much.

Drying Herbs

This quality can be felt on the tongue as you are tasting it. It can feel like a tightening on the tongue, a dry sensation after tasting the herb, or have a drying effect on the body. There are herbs that are slightly dry, some that are extremely dry, and some in-between. They help to tighten tissue, stop leakage, and draw out impurities. You will know what herbs fall into which category as you become more efficient in tasting, and when you develop more experiences with herbs. They tend to affect the kidneys, lungs, and skin or other tissue.

Drying herbs can stimulate fluid release, help to slow down fluid, or help in holding fluid in. These herbs can be considered astringent, expectorant, diuretic, diaphoretic, or hemostatic. They help to slow down bleeding, draw out infections, close wounds, tighten prolapsed organs, release phlegm, stimulate urine production, and sweat out toxins. In excess, these herbs could contribute to excessive dehydration and loss of electrolytes.

Moistening Herbs

The main purpose of moistening herbs is to nourish the tissue and the body. Herbs containing mucilage or oils are labeled moistening herbs. Since the body is made up of tissue, these herbs can affect the entire body depending on how they are taken either internally or externally.

Mucilage is a gelatinous constituent contained in herbs that is healing and can act as an expectorant, demulcent, emollient, or cell proliferant. They can help to break up phlegm or congestion, soothe irritated tissue, or help repair tissue. You will find they are beneficial for repairing connective tissue such as healing bones, tendons, or ligaments. They are also great to stimulate productive coughs, heal sore throats, soothe burns, or help with the elimination of the bowels. Mucilage-containing herbs could also slow down absorption of nutrients or pharmaceutical medications. It is best to take these herbs an hour before or after you consume food or take medications. Some of these herbs are tonics and excessive use would not be a problem; however, other moistening herbs could have individual side effects with larger doses. In this case, it is best to know the individual herb well.

Exercise

Create your own fire cider oxymel! There are a lot of versions using different herbs. Research each herb and experiment with different combinations or look up more recipes. The standard base includes garlic cloves, onions, horseradish, ginger root, and cayenne peppers. Other additions include citrus fruits of your choosing, rose hips, echinacea, cinnamon, turmeric, sweet leaf, basil, elderberries, etc. Chop up the herbs and layer in a mason jar. Fill organic apple cider vinegar in the jar to the top, cap (put barrier between metal lid and liquid), label, and shake daily for one month. Strain and add ¼–½ the volume with raw honey. Mix well.

Using your knowledge of taste, try adding different herbs to achieve the best flavor for you and your family! Make sure to journal each recipe so you don't forget what you used!

🌿 *You have now added another remedy to your apothecary!*

Chapter Seventeen
Human Energetics

Once you understand plant energetics, you can determine how they are matched to an individual by using human energetics. This includes utilizing the concept of both the human tissue states and an individual's constitution before moving forward in choosing the right herbs for each individual. First, I need to define what tissue states and constitutions are to you. You will have better chances of helping each person sooner and more successfully by doing it this way rather than choosing an herb based on their health conditions and symptoms only. By utilizing energetics, you can be a better herbalist. Keep in mind that the more you practice, the better you will become at noticing these energetic patterns and properly utilizing them.

Tissue States

Tissue states describe the condition of the tissue within the body. This can be determined by recognizing visual indicators, knowing the health conditions of an individual, or hearing cues given by the individual. Just as there are four qualities of plants, there are four qualities to humans too. However, they are referred to as tissue states instead. These tissue states are cold, hot, dry, and damp, tense and lax. Each of these tissue states can give the herbalist a good idea on the health of the individual, and what type of herbs will be needed to balance their body. You will notice that each tissue state has an opposite one. Keep this in mind as we move forward. When I describe each of the tissue states below, I will include what kind of assessments you might notice on the individual, what health conditions each could include, and what you might hear from the client as a clue to what tissue states are involved.

Cold

This tissue state is also referred to as Depression. A cold tissue state is often understood as a slowing of processes or reduction of activity. It could also represent a lack of response from the body. Slow digestion, lack of immune response, or slow circulation are some examples of a cold tissue state. You might notice the client is constipated, has cold hands or feet, you see a blue undertone in their skin, or notice that they are pale. These would be considered assessments which help the practitioner understand what is happening in the body. Cold tissue health conditions could include bloating and flatulence, hypothyroid or other hypo conditions, malnutrition, inactivity of organs, or a reduction in secretions from the body. Clues from the individual are important to listen for as indicators as well. They might state "I am moving slower in the mornings," "I am cold all the time," "I have lost so much energy," or "I have been experiencing brain fog lately."

Mary's Advice

Write down some health conditions that you or your family might have and describe the tissue states that correlate with them.

Hot

This tissue state is also referred to as Excitation. If a cold tissue state refers to the slowing of activity, a hot tissue state would refer to overactivity in the body. It could also be considered excess stimulation or hyperfunction. Visual assessments include visible redness on the skin, fidgeting, pain, or a red tongue. Health conditions with this tissue state could include inflammatory diseases, autoimmune diseases, high blood pressure or cholesterol, hyperthyroid, or Crohn's disease. The individual might state "I am always hot," "I am in pain all the time," "I'm out of control," or "I can't seem to slow down."

Dry

This tissue state is also referred to as Atrophy. Atrophy is the lack of fluid contributing to the wasting away of an organ or cells. Our body is made up of water and needs this water to sustain itself. If an individual continues to be dry, the cells wither away and do not function properly. The other way to look at dryness is a lack of oils in the body. This could be from a lack of healthy fats in the diet to a lack of oil secretions from the glands. You might also consider that this dryness isn't from a lack of fluids necessarily, but possibly from the loss of the ability to hold on to moisture or overheating of the system. Visual assessments could include dry skin, dry hair, dry scalp, cracks in the tongue, or lack of moisture on the tongue. Dry health conditions include constipation, dry mouth, cracking joints, degenerative diseases, excessive sweating, longstanding fevers, or sore throat. An individual might tell you "I not drinking much water," "My skin is dry and itchy," "My bowels are hard," or "I suffer from dry eyes."

Damp

This tissue state is also referred to as stagnation. Stagnation is the lack of fluid movement due to an accumulation of moisture or phlegm. This excess moisture blocks the elimination of fluid and absorption of nutrients, and it can restrict the delivery of secretions in the body. Visual assessments include a swollen or damp tongue, swelling anywhere in the body, rattling or wheezing in the lungs, puffy eyes or face, or sinus pressure. Health conditions include constant sinus infections or lung infections, edema, swollen lymph nodes, mucus in the stool, or kidney issues. The individual might mention "I have been coughing up mucus for a long time," "My feet swell every night," "I get a lot of infections," "I don't exercise or move much," or "I feel a heaviness in my body."

Tense

Also called constriction, this tissue state refers to the structure of the tissue being too tight. Excessive tight or tense tissue can be a contributor to the slowing down or restriction of movement. Constricted blood vessels can slow the movement of blood as an example. Tense muscles can also restrict movement of our body. It is easy to understand the implication of being too tense, and the need to balance it. Visual indicators are stiff movement, holding themselves too tightly, jaw clenching, anger episodes or frustration displayed, or raising of their voices. Health conditions associated with tense tissue state are irritable bowel syndrome, TMJ, tension headaches, nervousness, insomnia, restless legs syndrome, back and neck pain, or cramping. The individual could say "I cannot relax," "I am sore all of the time," "I grind my teeth at night," or "I feel angry all the time."

Lax

This tissue state, called atony, refers to a lack of tone in the structure of the tissue. Relaxed tone in the body releases more fluid, doesn't hold cell structure, and contributes to prolapsed organs. Laxity can create damp conditions by letting fluid through the tissue more easily where it can accumulate or cause dry conditions from the release of excess fluids. You can determine which condition the laxity is creating by looking at the other visual assessments in the individual or listening for other clues. Visual assessments could include sagging skin, dragging of the body when they walk, varicose veins, or bleeding gums. Health conditions could include incontinence, prolapsed organs, diarrhea, bleeding, or excessive perspiration. You might hear the individual say, "I leak urine when I jump," "Food just goes right through me," "I bleed easily," or "My veins are more prominent through my skin."

Constitutions

With human energetics, tissue states and the constitutional type of the individual are taken into consideration. Constitutions are basically a description of the person's physique or personality. Every traditional medical system calls them by different names and looks at various different aspects. In Ayurveda, they are called doshas, and in traditional Chinese medicine, they are called the nine body constitutions. The ancient Greeks introduced a system of the four humors of the body along with the four temperaments.

Because this subject can be somewhat confusing for the beginner, and for the sake of keeping this training simple, I will not be including detailed information about these. It is enough that you know it is considered along with tissue states when helping to choose the right herb for an individual. This knowledge is not necessary in order to finish this book, or to learn the basics of herbalism. Knowing the tissue states will be enough to start understanding the concept of energetics and how to balance the herb with the client. Training about constitutions should coincide with the traditional medical system that the student wishes to learn. It should be studied separately in a more detailed learning process to enhance the student's comprehension later, or with clinical training.

Chapter Eighteen
Combining Medicinal Properties and Energetics

In Chapter Eleven (page 49), we described the medicinal properties of herbs and how they acted on the body. In Chapter Fifteen (page 75), we explained what energetics were, and how they were divided into plant and human energetics. In this chapter, I want to explain how you use the knowledge from both to choose the right herb for an individual. There are multiple herbs containing the same medicinal properties, and all herbs can have multiple medicinal properties themselves. How do you decide which one to use? It is not based on the symptoms alone that the individual is experiencing. You look at the person first before choosing an herb.

Below, I am including simple steps to take in order to choose an herb to work with. I will describe how I handle each step so that you understand the concept.

1. **Determine the energetics of the individual with consideration of their tissue states.** I use the visual assessments, clues, and health conditions of the individual to determine what two tissue states they are experiencing at this moment.
2. **Determine what actions are needed in the body.** I consider primary and secondary concerns to determine what the individual needs to help with their immediate symptoms. Write down the main medicinal properties or actions you are looking for in an herb.
3. **Write down herbs that you have on hand that offer the needed actions.**
4. **Determine the plant energetics of each herb.** Refer back to Chapter Sixteen (page 78) for help if needed. You should also write each of these down under every herb on your list.

5. **Determine what plant energetics you need to balance the individual.** You want to look for the opposite quality. If the individual is both hot and dry, you want to balance them with a plant that is cool and moist.
6. **Cross off the herbs on your list that will not balance the individual.**
7. **Compare the herbs that are left on the list.** Which one has the most beneficial medicinal properties for this individual?
8. **Choose the herb.**

Sometimes you will need to choose more than one herb, but for the sake of this lesson, follow these steps before choosing an herb for each individual. Let's follow each step together with a fictional situation as an example:

A family member comes to me with a cough that has lasted for more than two weeks. They have not coughed up any phlegm. They are also experiencing nasal drip and a sore throat. Visually, I see that they have reddened cheeks, and they didn't come in with a coat in colder temperatures.

1. **I would say that this individual has hot and dry tissue states.** The reddened cheeks and the fact that they came in without a coat indicates the hot tissue state. The sore throat, no expectoration of mucus, and nasal drip indicates the dry tissue state because irritation and the loss of fluids could dry an individual out. Plus, the hot tissue state could further aggravate this dry tissue.
2. **This individual needs an expectorant to help cough up the phlegm, a demulcent to soothe the irritated tissue, and an astringent to stop the loss of fluid from the nasal cavity.**
3. **I know we haven't discussed herbs yet, but here are the ones I have on hand to choose from:**
   a. Marshmallow root (*Althaea officinalis*)
   b. Self-heal (*Prunella vulgaris*)
   c. Hyssop (*Hyssopus officinalis*)
   d. Mullein (*Verbascum thapsus*)
4. **I have determined the energetics of each herb:**
   a. Marshmallow: cool and moist

    b. Self-heal: cool and moist

    c. Hyssop: warm and dry

    d. Mullein: cool and moist

5. **I am looking for a cool and moist herb to balance the hot and dry tissue states of the individual.**

6. **I will cross off hyssop from my list because it is not cool and moist.**

7. **Only one of the herbs left on the list has all three medicinal properties I need.** The other two are both expectorants and demulcents but are not considered astringents.

8. **The herb I would choose is self-heal.** It is considered a cooling and moistening expectorant, demulcent, and astringent.

With continued practice and a better knowledge of herbs, you will become efficient at choosing the right herb for an individual. Novice herbalists do not usually consider energetics when they choose an herb. They would have chosen mullein leaves or marshmallow root for the cough just because they know they are considered expectorants and used for coughs. They do not first consider what kind of cough it is (moist or dry), or the individual's tissue states. They choose an herb based on their symptoms or conditions only. Knowing about energetics sets you up as a successful herbalist in the future.

Exercise

Choose five people experiencing different symptoms around you. Use the information in the previous chapters to determine the individual's energetics. Then determine the medicinal properties needed, and the plant energetics needed to balance these individuals. Keep this list because you will return to it after learning about herbs in Chapter Twenty-One (page 102).

PART FIVE

Introduction to Herbs

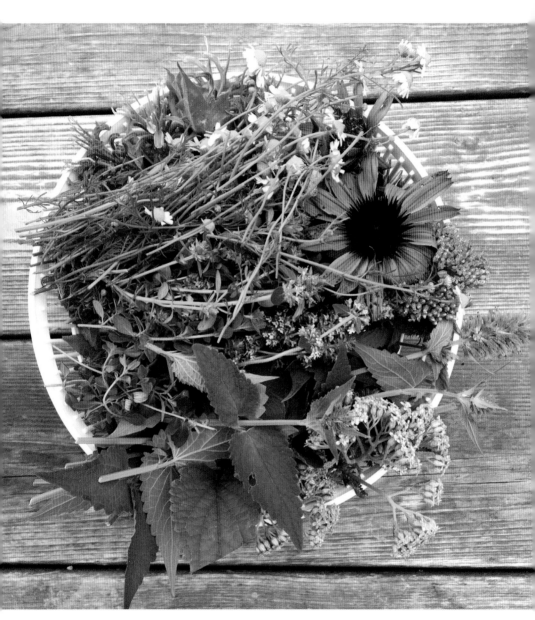

© Denise Cusack

Chapter Nineteen
How to Use This Section

Congratulations on getting to this part of the book! You now have a solid foundation of understanding herbalism and are ready to begin learning about individual herbs. You need to first understand the basic medicinal properties, energetics, harvesting basics, and the types of herbal preparations before researching and learning about individual herbs so that you understand the information you are reading. You can learn what each herb does for the body but eventually confusion will set in while you are studying each one if you haven't studied these basics first. You will be distracted by looking up some of this information that you don't understand, which can lead to becoming overwhelmed. I want to help you avoid all of that. That is why I have laid out the steps of this book this way.

Mary's Advice

I always advise my students to study five herbs at a time and learn everything they can about them. Research all five herbs individually, grow them, or make medicine with each to experience and connect with it fully. Don't try to just memorize information. Once you feel confident about those five herbs, you can move on to learn more.

I am including thirty-five herbs in this book for you to study and get hands-on experience with. These herbs will be used to set up your home apothecary to help yourself, your family, and your friends. They are laid out alphabetically so that you can use Chapter Twenty-One (page 102) as a quick reference in the future when needed.

Mary's Advice

If you are studying these herbs in the off-growing season, you can purchase the herb from a reputable source. Check the next chapter for ideas on where to get your herbs.

I will mention the taste, qualities, parts used, and the medicinal properties of each herb. Additionally, I will include the different herbal preparations that can be used, and how I have utilized each in my experience and practice. It is my hope that you will do some further research about each herb including its history or folklore, any modern scientific studies with the herb, its identification and growing conditions, and much more before doing the exercises. Check the contraindications and interactions especially if you or anyone else has a health condition or are currently on any pharmaceutical medications before taking any herb internally. Please refer to the disclaimer at the beginning of this book before using any of these herbal preparations and formulas. Safety is first.

With each herb, I will include an exercise to give you hands-on experience making medicine with it. Remember the journals that you started in prior exercises? It would be a good idea for you to keep a journal about the herb as you make medicine with it and taste each one (keeping safety in mind). Document how you made your medicine, what it tasted like, how it worked in your body, and what dose you took. Feel free to try other herbal preparations based on your research. In a perfect scenario, you can see these herbs in person, harvest from them directly, make medicine with their parts, and use the medicine yourself; however, this is not always possible. Do the best you can and have fun doing it!

Exercise

Harvest or purchase each of the thirty-five herbs prior to working with them in the Chapter Twenty-One exercises (page 102). Work at your own pace due to finances, seasons, or availability of the herbs in your area.

Chapter Twenty
Herbal Resources

As an herbalist, one of the most important things to consider is where to first obtain the herbs before making the medicine for the apothecary. This all depends on the area the herbalist lives in, the climate they reside in, what type of access they have for harvesting herbs, what the availability of an herb is in their area, what kind of access to community farmers or other herbalists they have, or their current finances. Again, not all herbalists are the same, and some might have different ideas on the best way to resource their herbs.

You have already obtained the herbs used in this book by purchasing them online, harvesting them, or even growing some of them yourself. It's even possible you were able to find a local farmer or herbalist near you and purchase the herbs from them. I want to share with you my thoughts on the best resources for obtaining herbs for medicine and the reasons for my opinions.

When we moved to our new house and land, I knew that I needed to get my gardens going first thing. My vegetable garden was my first priority alongside a small garden for herbs near the office. I have also taken the time to document what herbs or trees are present on the property along with the amounts of each. I do this because I like to harvest my medicine directly from the source if I can and have my herbs as fresh as possible for future processing. I like to make a list of what is currently growing around me, what I can grow in the future, and what herbs I will be needing to purchase for my business.

I want to offer my favorite resources for supplying your apothecary in the order I like to follow:

1. **Grow your own**. I love to grow and harvest my own herbs if I have the space available first and foremost! This allows for the herbs to be collected as fresh as possible and used immediately or dried for later use. It also assures that my herbs are given the correct nutrients,

are organic as possible, and thrive under my supervision and love. I prefer this resource over the next simply because I don't want to take much from the wild if I don't have to.

2. **Wildcraft or forage around your area**. Make sure to follow the harvesting rules with this and make sure you harvest sustainably. This resource also allows my herbs to be collected as fresh as possible, which is why it is number two.

3. **Local farmers or herb growers**. I am currently gathering a list for myself and others around me with local businesses that grow and harvest herbs to sell. You can often get the herbs fresh for pick-up, or dried herbs can be shipped if needed. This is another way to get the herbs as fresh as possible if you do not personally grow or have this herb growing in your area.

4. **Other herbalists**. This is another great option to use if the first three are not possible. If the herbalist grew or harvested the herb from their area, you will also have a fresh source of quality herbs. I have asked and paid herbalists from other states to ship me what they have harvested because it doesn't grow in my area, or the local growers are sold out of my choices of herbs.

5. **Herbal suppliers**. This is my last choice because it is often more expensive, they have to heat-treat their herbs to sanitize them here in the United States, and they are often sold out of herbs because so many people utilize this resource first.

For me, the best resource is the option where I can harvest and process my herbs immediately. If you cannot harvest immediately yourself and have to purchase the herbs, the time between harvesting and processing of the herbs needs to be considered due to shipping or even the time it was stored on a shelf. You can ask the herb grower or herbalist when their harvesting time was or get the lot number where you can call the supplier for the harvesting date of the herb(s).

There are times when I need an herb in a hurry for one of my clients. If I do not have enough here on my shelves or I cannot harvest the herb currently, I will have to purchase the herb. My client might not be able to wait for shipping so I will visit a health food store in my area that sells bulk herbs. I do not have any local herb shops near me. I check the lot numbers in this case and ask the shop when this herb was purchased by them. They can usually check when it was purchased, or you can call the company that supplied them with the lot number to find the age. Any herb harvested within a year is good, but longer than that could contribute to a quality issue with the herb.

Exercise

In this exercise, you will create a journal of herbs that you are growing, herbs that are growing around you, and herbs that you need for your apothecary in the future. Using the future herbs needed in your apothecary, decide on where you will resource them.

Chapter Twenty-One
The Herbs

The herbs that are included in this chapter grow in my area of Northern Ohio in the United States of America. I live near the Vermilion River and its tributaries, which have carved into this landscape for over ten thousand years.[13] Native and non-native species are prevalent here. Many of these herbs have different varieties of the same species growing elsewhere in the world. Research what plants are available in your area specifically and how they can be used medicinally if you cannot find the individual herb that I mention here growing near you. When you are researching each herb, look at where the plant is naturalized and introduced to see if it grows near you. Also, look into what hardiness zones they grow in and the specific growing conditions they need if you are wanting to wild harvest or grow them yourself. You can buy herbs if they are not available or look into researching other herbs with the same energetics and medicinal properties around you as alternative herbs in your medicine chest.

Mary's Advice

Take a look through the herbs in this chapter and write down the ones that you are familiar with. Choose the five herbs out of this list to begin learning.

As you are studying, make sure you are taking the time to enjoy what you are learning and as the old saying goes, "Stop and smell the roses!" Use all of your senses to experience each one of these herbs if you can. This is not a numbers game with knowing the most herbs. This is a journey to connecting with our plant allies.

Black walnut (*Juglans nigra*)

Taste: Bitter

Qualities: Warming and drying

Parts used: Hulls, inner bark, leaves, root

Medicinal properties: Alterative, anthelmintic, antifungal, antimicrobial, antiphlogistic (anti-inflammatory), astringent, cholagogue, cathartic, digestive, hepatic, sialagogue

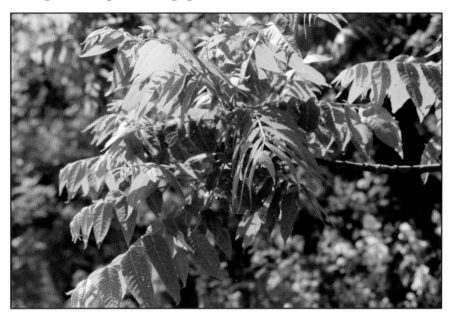

Black walnut trees are known for the strength of their wood, but they are also considered to be strong medicine. Every part of this tree is used in herbalism including the roots, leaves, hulls, bark, and walnuts. The walnuts are very nutritious with a multitude of health benefits (if you succeed in extracting them from the shell). My grandfather used his car to break the nut from the shell because they are so hard to crack. Nutcrackers will not do the job easily. The inner bark and leaves can be considered between an aperient and a purgative depending on the dosage used. Smaller internal doses are aperient, while larger internal doses can be purgative. Almost every part of the tree is considered anthelmintic, antimicrobial, antifungal, anti-inflammatory, astringent, and digestive. The bitter taste is contained in all parts of the tree and contributes towards the sialagogue, cholagogue, and hepatic medicinal properties.

I prefer to use the leaves and the hulls only in my practice due to the efficiency of harvesting, and the sheer number of trees available to me. I will dry the leaves for use in infusions, ointments, and fomentations. I will also harvest the fresh hulls from the ground (with gloves) once they start turning black, but still have some green coloring to them, and immediately make a fresh tincture. I either use drop dosing or standard dosing with this herb.

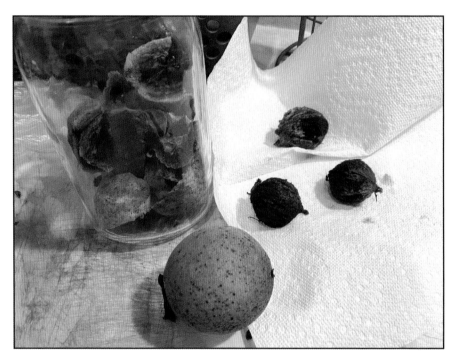

Black walnut leaves make a great addition to any external application for skin issues, fungal infections, ringworm, varicose veins, or small wounds. They also work very well to reduce swelling in connective tissue. A warm infusion of the leaves will make a good wash externally, or an addition to a bath for fungal infections or hemorrhoids. Internally, either the warm infusion of the leaves or the tincture of the hulls can be taken for parasitic infections, stimulating the digestive system, toning tissue, or for reducing inflammation. It is often utilized in the south as a remedy for both hyperthyroidism (goiters) and hypothyroidism.[14] In *The Practicing Herbalist*, Margi Flint uses black walnut hulls as an herb specifically for the adrenals.[15]

Exercise

Collect or purchase the leaves of black walnut and make this simple warm infusion to help you understand the process of infusing with herbs. You will use:

1 ounce dried black walnut leaves, a large infuser, a pan, and 4 cups distilled water

Place the herb in an infuser (standard measurements are 1 ounce herb to 1 cup water, but these leaves are very lightweight, so I often don't measure and just fill the infuser). Fill a pan with the water and place the infuser in the water. Bring the water to a boil, then reduce to a simmer, cover with a lid, and let the herb steep in the water for 15 to 20 minutes. For a stronger infusion, steep for 40 to 60 minutes. Remove the infuser. (Some herbs steep overnight depending on the herb or the property needed. Research each herb for this information.) You can use this warm infusion in your bathtub or footbath for antifungal, antimicrobial, or astringent benefits or drink internally (always research and check contraindication/interactions first).

🌿 You have added a potent herb to your apothecary to make more medicine as needed!

Burdock (*Arctium lappa, A. minus*)

Taste: Slightly sweet, salty, and bitter

Qualities: Cooling and moistening

Parts used: Leaves, root, seeds, stalk

Medicinal properties: Alterative, antiphlogistic, demulcent, depurative, diuretic, digestive, emollient, hepatic, lymphatic, nutritive, and tonic

My grandfather told me stories about how his family would collect the stalks from the second-year plant, peel the rind, and boil the stalk in order to eat them. He said they were delicious and very nutritious. Another nutritious food source from burdock is the root. In Japan, it is called gobo and added to soups, sushi rolls, and other culinary treats. The root and leaves contain mucilage and are considered demulcent and emollient, which soothe the tissue of the body both internally and externally. All parts of the plant are bitter tasting; and therefore, contribute a hepatic and depurative action on the body. The roots and seeds are diuretic with the seeds more pronounced in that property. The alterative property from burdock comes from increasing function in both the lymphatic and digestive systems. It also helps in the metabolism of lipids (fats) in the body.

You want to harvest the root in the first year of growth since this plant is a biennial. It forms the leaves in the first year, and the stalk and

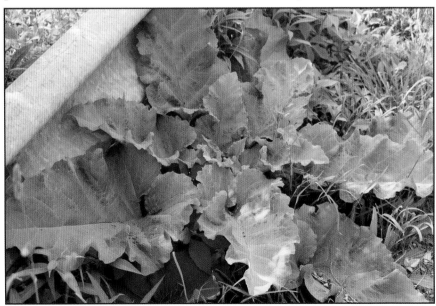

flowers in the second year. Once it flowers, it reseeds and dies back, leaving the seedlings to start the cycle again. I utilize the root mostly in my practice, but I do use the leaves at times for its emollient and demulcent properties. I like to dry the root for use in infusions and decoctions and make a fresh or dried root tincture for convenience and a longer shelf life. I usually start with a lower dose and increase the amount of medicine as needed. Sometimes the smaller doses of this herb work better than the larger doses. This is, of course, dependent on the situation.

The root medicine is often used to benefit skin conditions such as acne, psoriasis, or eczema. It is also good at moving the eliminatory channels to detoxify. This includes the liver, kidneys, lymph nodes, and skin. I choose burdock when I need to balance a dry and hot condition, when there is systemic imbalance or inflammation, or the endocrine system needs nourished or balanced.

Exercise

In this exercise, you will use dried burdock root to make a decoction. You will use:

1 ounce dried burdock root, a large infuser with a lid, a pan, and 4 cups distilled water

Place the dried root in the infuser and put the lid on. Fill the pan with the water and place the infuser in the water (or add root in the water and strain afterward). Bring the water to a boil, then reduce to a simmer, cover, and continue to simmer for 20 minutes. Take off the heat and leave it covered while it steeps for another 20 minutes. Remove the infuser.

Take the opportunity here to taste the decoction in small sips at a time. Get to know how this herb is acting on your body. Close your eyes and track its progress. Save the rest for additional doses during the day. Record your results in your journal.

🌿 You have just added another beneficial herb to your medicine chest! More remedies will be made with this herb later!

Calendula (*Calendula officinalis*)

Taste: Bitter, pungent, and somewhat sweet

Qualities: Warming and drying with a cooling aftereffect

Parts used: Flowering head (ray) that includes many individual flowers

Medicinal properties: Alterative, antifungal, antiphlogistic, antiseptic, astringent, cell proliferant, cholagogue, digestive, emmenagogue, lymphatic, sialagogue, vulnerary

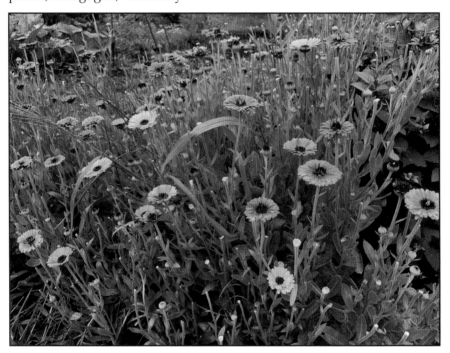

© Denise Cusack

Calendula is an easy-to-grow plant no matter what type of housing or community you live in. The flowerheads are utilized in both internal and external applications medicinally using multiple types of herbal preparations. You will get more flower production to harvest if the flowers are removed often. They do contain larger amounts of volatile oils and resins that are better extracted in oils or alcohol to get the most potency but are still viable in a warm infusion if the steeped herb is covered to prevent the loss of the volatile oils.

I grow my calendula in raised beds, and I will also be adding them to some of my new gardens soon. As stated before, I pick the flowers as soon as they open to help with further flower production. The flowers take a little longer to dry than some other herbs due to their density. Make sure they are completely dried before you seal them away in a jar. I will make an infusion, tincture, oil, and ointment with calendula. I will also add them to foot baths or warm baths, use them as a fomentation, or combine them with other herbs in a formula. This is an herb that can be used in larger doses up to four milliliters three times daily in a tincture, or up to six cups daily based on the needs of an individual. You can follow drop doses, standard doses, or maximum doses of this herb according to the situation.

I consider calendula a "sunny herb," meaning it will help someone feeling "down in the dumps" or a bit depressed. I have used it in cases of seasonal affective disorder with good results. Calendula is also good in cases of excess candida overgrowth either used internally or externally. The warm infusion, oil, or ointment is beneficial externally for many different medicinal actions including healing wounds, drawing out infections, reducing swollen tissue and glands, and reducing bleeding. I like to add them to baths for fungal infections, healing of tissue, and as a general drying agent for any weeping sores.

Exercise

In this exercise, you will use dried calendula flower heads in a warm bath or foot bath. If you do not have a bathtub or footbath, you can use a large bowl or pot to soak your foot or feet in. You will need: A large muslin bag, enough calendula flowers to fill it (you can also add Epsom salts and some chamomile flowers to this if you prefer).

Fill the muslin bag with the herb(s) and tie it closed. Tie the bag around the faucet of the tub and let the warm water run through it for a bit, then throw it in the water to steep.

You can also make a warm infusion in larger batches and pour it in the tub or footbath (or bowl/pot).

You made a bolus earlier with this herb, and now you will have multiple opportunities to use this herb and create other formulas in this book for your apothecary!

Chamomile (*Matricaria chamomilla*)

Taste: Bitter

Qualities: Slightly warm to cooling (Neutral) and drying

Parts used: Flowers

Medicinal properties: Anodyne, anthelmintic, antiphlogistic, antispas-modic, carminative, cathartic (large doses), diaphoretic, digestive, emetic (large doses), emmenagogue, hepatic, nervine, sedative

Chamomile is one of those herbs that a lot of people are familiar with. It is a standard remedy as a sedative herb, and it is often found as a simple tea in the grocery aisle. The flow-ers produce all of the above medicinal properties, but they are prepared in different ways depending on the actions that are needed. As a tonic emmen-agogue, a cold infusion would need to be prepared. If the dia-phoretic property is needed, a warm infusion will need to be taken while it is hot. If you

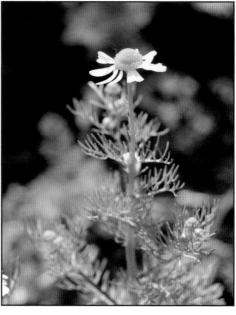

need more of the bitter taste to come through, you would steep it for longer in an infusion (or make a tincture). A poultice, oil, or ointment made with the flowers will act as an antispasmodic, relaxing nervine, or antiphlogistic. Using the fresh flowers in either a tincture or an infusion will bring out more of the relaxing properties than dried flowers.

For flower production, I pick the flowers as soon as they open to promote more growth and harvest opportunities. If you do not pick the flowers, they will reseed and spread all over the area. I will often dry the flowers to store for use throughout the year, or use the fresh flowers in my infusions, tinctures, and glycerites to be made during the grow-ing season. I like to include chamomile flowers in cosmetics, oils and ointments, bath soaks, infusions, glycerites, and tinctures. Drop dosing to standard dosing is often utilized with this herb.

This herb is invaluable to me as a gentle sedative or stimulating digestive for younger children used in correct doses for their weight. I also like to add it to my lotions or creams to help reduce puffiness and redness, and to relieve tension. I will often combine chamomile with other herbs in specific formulas for my clients for their digestive, nervine, or hepatic needs. Of course, I use the flowers in my baths to help in reducing spasms, and for aromatherapy to relax. I find it indicated for the individual that is "hot under the collar," so to speak, or keeps their anger just under the surface, that is in need of some relaxation and more time to enjoy the better things in life.

Exercise

In this exercise, you will be making different variations of an infusion. Make a warm infusion with 1 cup boiling water poured over approximately ¼ ounce flowers, cover, and let steep for 10 minutes, then make a second infusion exactly the same way but steep for 30 minutes. Taste the difference and feel the effects in your body. Add the findings to your journal. Did you taste a difference or feel different actions in the body?

The second step to this exercise is to make a warm infusion with fresh flowers when available and one with dried flowers. Document the taste and actions felt within your body. Did you feel any differences or similarities?

🍃 The endless applications of this one herb will benefit your apothecary and help you create more remedies when needed.

Chickweed (*Stellaria media*)

Taste: Sweet

Qualities: Cooling and moistening

Parts used: Herb (everything above the ground)

Medicinal properties: Alterative, antiphlogistic, aperient, astringent, demulcent, depurant, diuretic, emollient, expectorant, lymphatic, nutritive, vulnerary

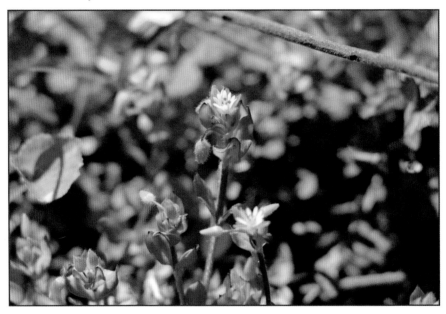

Chickweed is one of the first herbs you will find in the springtime and is considered a spring tonic. A spring tonic is an herb that contains nutrients and stimulates the digestive and lymphatic systems to encourage elimination. It is sweet tasting and very nutritious, which many of the green plants growing in the spring are considered. I have an area by the stream that is abundant in chickweed, and they are often found in disturbed areas. Harvest the aerial herb according to the harvesting rules. You will want to make sure you have more to harvest for the years ahead. The aerial portions of the herb are responsible for all the above medicinal properties. Chickweed contains a good amount of mucilage, which has been previously mentioned as contributing to the demulcent, emollient, and expectorant properties.

I harvest the edible fresh aerial parts for both culinary and medicinal purposes. It includes a good source of proteins and minerals. I like to include this herb when I make a salad, smoothie, or pesto. I also make infusions, tinctures, oils, ointments, and baths using this herb. It is best to cut the herb up before placing it in your salads or soups because of the inside fibrous cord located further down the stem. The best way to identify and know you have *S. media* is to locate the single line of hairs on one side of the stem. Other varieties of chickweed do not have this particular feature. I utilize the standard dosing philosophy when I recommend it.

Chickweed has been traditionally used to help people with weight loss, and science has recently confirmed this.[16] I will consider recommending this herb internally using either food or with other herbal preparations to some of my clients with a slower metabolism or nutrient deficiencies. I also like to add chickweed to baths and infuse my oils and ointments to help soothe dry, itchy skin or eruptions. I also recommend chickweed as a gentle lymph stimulant along with movement when there is congestion in the lymphatic system. I look at chickweed as an all-around gentle alterative that almost everyone can benefit from as food, medicine, or both.

Exercise

In this exercise, I want you to harvest some fresh local chickweed if it is available to you and find a way to use it in your diet. Experiment and taste the herb. Which way do you like it best?

If you cannot find any chickweed around you or you wish to do another herbal preparation, use the dried herb to make an infused lymph massage oil. You will need: Double boiler pans, 1½ cups olive oil, approximately ½ ounce dried chickweed, cheesecloth, a strainer, large glass measuring cup, bottle with cap, and label.

Add water to the bottom of your double boiler and the olive oil and herb in the top pan. Bring the water to a gentle boil and simmer for an hour, stirring occasionally. Place the cheesecloth over a strainer and place the strainer on a large glass measuring cup. Pour the infused oil into the cheesecloth-covered strainer and let the oil drain. Squeeze out any excess liquid, let it cool down, then bottle and cap it. Label and store in a cool, dark cabinet.

🌿 *This oil base has now been added to your apothecary with other uses!*

Cleavers (*Galium aparine*)

Taste: Sweet, salty, and slightly bitter with a metallic aftertaste

Qualities: Cooling and moistening

Parts used: Herb

Medicinal properties: Alterative, antioxidant, antiphlogistic, aperient, astringent, diuretic, lymphatic, tonic

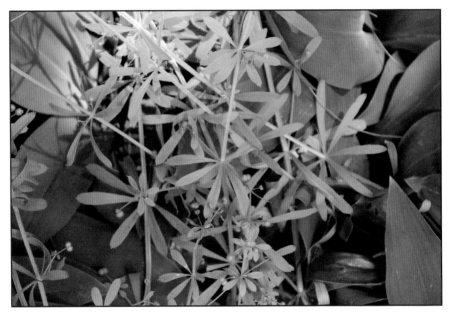

© Denise Cusack

Cleavers is another springtime herb that offers vitamins and minerals with a high vitamin C content; and therefore, produces antioxidant activities. As a child, I would throw them on my brother's back just to have him notice them later on in the day. It was fun to watch them stick to clothing due to the small hooks covering the plant. It was even more fun when he discovered them there later on! When you boil the herb, these tiny hooks soften and are unnoticeable when eaten. The whole herb is used medicinally to produce all of the properties above.

I collect the herb as soon as I see the very tiny white flowers opening and take them home to juice for a succus. I will then add alcohol to this as a preservative. I will also dry the herb thoroughly for later use in either infusions or oils and ointments. The plant contains a lot of moisture and should be dried completely with good air flow before sealing it in a jar. The fresh flowers can be made into a succus, infusion, or tincture while the dried flowers work best in either an infusion or made into an oil. I like to use drop to standard doses, and I will use for longer periods of time if needed.

Cleavers is a traditional herb for the lymphatic system and for the kidneys. It is a powerful alterative moving the lymph system and for urinary output. It is also beneficial as a gentle laxative when the bowels aren't moving efficiently. Interestingly enough, cleavers will also benefit diarrhea due to its astringent property. Inflammation in the kidneys, urinary tract, or prostate is cooled and soothed while the herb contributes to the proper functioning of each. I personally like to use it mostly in a succus herbal preparation as a tonic for the lymph and urinary system. Although, I do like to make an oil or ointment with cleavers combined with violet leaves and flowers as a lymph massage, or to benefit the individual in cases of fibrocystic breasts or breast cancer. I also like to include a fresh tincture if my clients need cleavers added to their formulas.

Exercise

For this exercise, you will use fresh cleavers to make a succus, or you can freeze the juice for later use throughout the year.

For the succus you will need: A juicer or blender, harvested fresh cleavers, distilled water, 195 proof grain alcohol, jar or bottle, and a label. You could also use a food processor or mortar and pestle to mash the herb thoroughly.

If you have a juicer or blender, just collect the juice. If not, simply add a little distilled water to the herb, mash, place the mashed herb in some cheesecloth, and squeeze or press out the juice.

Once the juice is collected, add the alcohol in a ratio of 3:1 which is 3 parts of the juice to 1 part alcohol. Let this sit for three days, then re-strain the liquid.

🌿 Add this succus to your apothecary!

Comfrey (*Symphytum officinale*)

Taste: Bland and slightly sweet
Qualities: Cooling and moistening
Parts used: Leaves and root
Medicinal properties: Anodyne, astringent, cell proliferant, demulcent, emollient, expectorant, hemostatic, nutritive, vulnerary

I studied from the teachings of Dr. Christopher when I began my own journey into herbalism. He used comfrey in a lot of his formulas, and I have used it often enough to know this herb works well in many of the properties above. Over the years, studies have shown that comfrey contains Pyrrolizidine alkaloids (PAs), which can cause hepatic veno-occlusive disease (VOD) when taken internally.[17] Most of the PAs are contained in the root with less in the leaves and flowers, and *S. officinale* contains less than Russian comfrey (*S. x uplandicum*).[18] This has led to a ban of the outright commercial sale of this herb for internal use here in the United States, and has inspired debate in the herbal community over internal consumption. As a clinical herbalist, it is my job to keep safety uppermost in my mind for my clients, which is why I use other alternative herbs medicinally for internal use, and I only use this herb in external applications when needed. I believe everyone should research

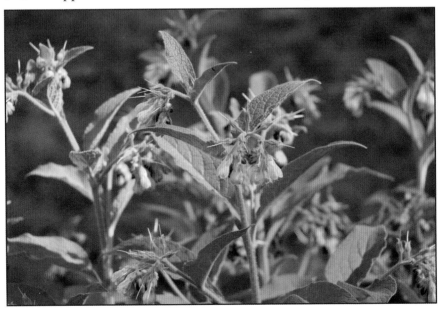

this herb thoroughly and base their practice on what feels right for them personally.

I will harvest both the root in the fall, and the leaves with flowers as soon as the flowers open. Both are interchangeable with similar actions. I like to make an oil or decoction containing comfrey root for external uses and the leaves internally in an infusion.

Comfrey has a long tradition as a soothing demulcent and emollient; as well as an expectorant and cell proliferant. This herb is beneficial for reducing swellings, healing connective tissue including bones, reducing pain associated with broken bones or sprains, healing burns, soothing rashes and itchy skin, and healing wounds. I have used it for all the previous mentioned mainly in an oil or fomentation. I used to utilize it as an expectorant, but I have found just as good alternative herbs for that need. Caution is warranted if you have a deep wound since comfrey closes the wound quickly, and therefore, could seal an infection inside.

Exercise

For this exercise, you will use the dried root to make a decoction and use it as a fomentation externally. You will need 4 cups distilled water, 1 ounce dried comfrey root, and a saucepan with a lid.

Place the distilled water and the root in the saucepan and bring it to a boil. Once boiling, reduce the heat and simmer for 20 minutes. Take off the heat, put on the lid, and steep for another 20 minutes. Strain the herb and let the decoction cool just a bit so it doesn't burn you.

Dip a cotton cloth (I use unbleached cotton diapers) into the decoction and squeeze out the excess. Place externally on an area in need and cover with another towel or plastic wrap to help contain the heat. This is a moist heat application to deliver the properties of the herb.

🌿 This first aid herb will benefit your apothecary in the future!

Dandelion (*Taraxacum officinale*)

Taste: Bitter and salty

Qualities: Cooling and drying

Parts used: Flower, leaves, and root

Medicinal properties: Alterative, antiphlogistic, antispasmodic, aperient, cholagogue, diuretic, hepatic, nutritive, sialagogue

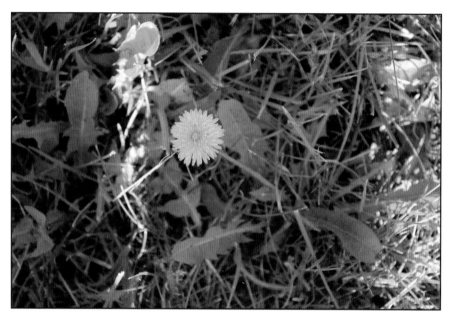

© Denise Cusack

Most people look at dandelion as a pest in the lawn while herbalists and nutritionists recognize the benefits they provide. It's a common herb and easily obtainable as long as there are no chemicals used on or around them. You can find the leaves in the produce section of the grocery store or the roots at a health food store or online. I believe the leaves produce more diuretic and nutritive actions on the body than the root does, and the root is more potent on the liver and gallbladder; however, all parts of the plant help the kidneys, liver, and gallbladder medicinally. The flowers are edible and used to make wine, infuse vinegars, or flavor beer for antioxidants and nutrition.

I like to pick the young leaves in the spring to add them to my salads or make an infused vinegar along with the flowers as a digestive and a nutritive. I also blanch and freeze the leaves for nutrition for the winter and add them to my soups and stir-fries. I make dandelion wine using the fresh flowers every year. I harvest the roots in the fall to make a fresh tincture and cut and dry them for use during the rest of the year. Most of this dried root is used to make ointments or decoctions for myself, my family, and my clients. Dosing is usually standard.

I like to combine dandelion with other herbs in my practice when I need hepatic, diuretic, and digestive properties. I will also use this herb to help stimulate the appetite if needed. With almost every known vitamin and mineral, dandelion is a good choice to add to your diet for nutritional benefits. At times, I will suggest the use of the latex from the stem to help in the removal of a wart, but I find that taxing since it takes using it consistently for weeks before it works.

Exercise

In this exercise, I want you to use fresh dandelion flowers and leaves to make your own infused vinegar. If not now, then once they become available. (You can make an infusion of the leaves or a decoction of the roots to taste and record in your journal if it is not that time of year yet for you.)

You will need: Fresh dandelion flowers and leaves, a pint jar with lid, organic apple cider vinegar, wax paper, and a label.

Cut the flowers and leaves, wash them thoroughly, and pack the jar with them. Fill the jar with apple cider vinegar, place wax paper over the jar, cap it, and label it. Let this macerate for 4 to 6 weeks on your counter. Shake daily, then strain when the time is up. Store this vinegar in a cooler, dark area out of direct sunlight. This does not need to be refrigerated and can last 3 to 6 months.

🍃 *Keep this herb and vinegar handy in your apothecary for both food and medicine!*

Echinacea (*Echinacea* spp.)

Taste: Sweet with a bitter aftertaste and tingling sensation (diffusive)

Qualities: Cold and drying

Parts used: Flower, leaf, and root

Medicinal properties: Alterative, analgesic, anodyne, antiphlogistic, antiseptic, antivenomous, depurant, immune-modulating, lymphatic, sialagogue

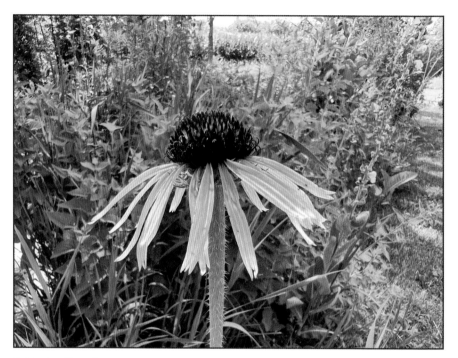

© Denise Cusack

There are many different species of Echinacea growing in North America with similar and interchangeable medicinal properties. It is commonly known as an immune stimulant for colds and flus, but in actuality, it is an immune modulator.[19] Traditionally, it was used to prevent sepsis and putrefaction, and used as a remedy for snake bites, which is different from how it is commonly used today for the immune system. All parts of the herb can provide the medicinal properties mentioned above. I find the root more diffusive (tingling), which might indicate a little more potency, but that is just my take on it. This is a good herb to use as an

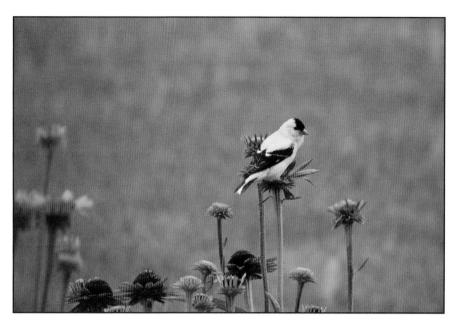

© Denise Cusack

example of the differences between traditional and modern medicinal usage and is a good reason to study the historical use of different herbs as well as modern science.

The leaves can be harvested from plants that are over two years old, and used either fresh or dried for infusions, vinegars, tinctures, glycerites, poultices, or fomentations. The roots can be harvested in the fall after they reach two years of age as well. I make a fresh tincture or glycerite with these, and then dry the rest for later use. All echinacea species are considered at-risk herbs with the United Plant Savers and should not be harvested from the wild. Echinacea is easily grown in the garden and spreads easily if you leave the flower heads on the plant to overwinter. They also make a good food source for birds at this time. Dosing with echinacea depends on the need, and can be dosed anywhere from drop dosing to maximum dosing. This is not an herb that you take for long periods of time. I was taught to take it for seven days and give the body a break from it for a day or two, and then resume only if needed, which is a form of pulse dosing.

I like to use the tincture and glycerite and add the fresh leaves or roots to fire cider or bone broth for immune support. I mostly combine echinacea in formulas rather than using it as a simple for alterative, decongestant, and analgesic properties. Dr. Christopher stated, "It is excellent wherever tissue decay is imminent or taking place, repair power is poor, and where there are unhealthy or bloody-tinged discharges."[20] I will use the maximum dosage for long-standing infections, when wounds are not healing (internal use), and for boils or infected cysts (internally and externally).

Exercise

For this exercise, you will make your first tincture using the folk medicine technique.

You will need: 1 pint- or quart-sized jar, dried echinacea root, 100 proof vodka (unflavored), and a label.

Fill half of the jar with the dried root, then pour the vodka to the top. Cap and label with the name of the herb, the date it was made, and the alcohol content (100 proof alcohol is 50 percent alcohol content). Shake it daily and leave it to macerate for 4 weeks. Strain, then store in a cool, dark cabinet.

🌿 Congratulations on adding the first tincture to your apothecary! (Mark in your journal how much alcohol content you used to make a dried tincture of echinacea for future reference.)

Elder (*Sambucus* spp.)

Taste: Sweet and sour

Qualities: Cool and somewhat drying

Parts used: Berries, flowers

Medicinal properties: Alterative, antioxidant, antiphlogistic, antispasmodic, antiviral, aperient, astringent, demulcent, diaphoretic, diuretic, emollient, expectorant, immunostimulant

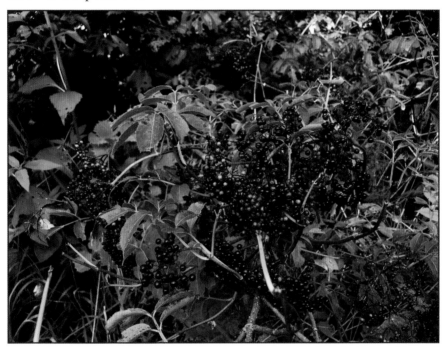

© Denise Cusack

Elderberry syrup is a popular and trending herbal preparation that you can find almost anywhere; however, it was the flowers that were traditionally used at the onset of a cold or flu when a fever persisted and the body wouldn't cool down. The diaphoretic property is achieved in a warm infusion using the flowers or berries, and it needs to be ingested while it is still warm to produce this action in the body. By stimulating perspiration, the body can cool down and eliminate toxins and waste. A cold infusion of the flowers will provide stronger demulcent, emollient, and expectorant properties to help soothe irritated tissue such as a sore throat or inflamed nasal cavities. Both the flowers and the berries offer immune support and antiviral activity, but the flowers are more astringent than the berries and can help with reducing nasal drip due to colds or allergies. The berries are sour tasting and produce a stronger diuretic property than the flowers.

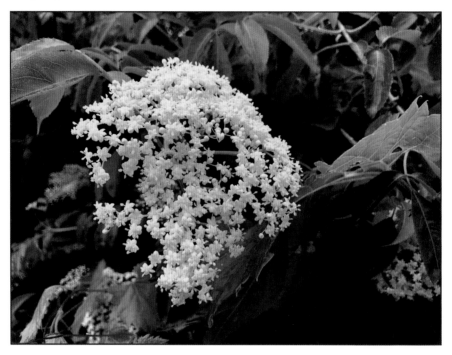

© Denise Cusack

The flowers are harvested in the early summer as soon as they open. I cut individual umbels and dry them before shaking and removing the individual flowers. The berries are harvested in the autumn if you can get to them before the birds do. You can cover the shrubs with netting if you grow them in your garden. I tend to reach for the flowers more often in my practice than I do the berries. Personally, I don't choose to use elderberry syrup as my go-to herbal preparation for the immune system due to the amount of sugar content it contains. I use tinctures or infusions mostly. Standard doses are used with this herb.

The flowers can be used when the immune system needs extra support, if an individual needs the benefits of a good sweat, or if a reduction in nasal and sinus congestion is needed. I mostly like combining elderflowers or berries with other herbs in a blend to expectorate mucus and reduce inflammation, to alleviate cramping in the digestive system, or to soothe a urinary tract infection.

Exercise

Get ready to make a glycerite formula that includes dried elderflowers.

You will need: Dried elderflowers, yarrow flowers, peppermint leaves, a quart jar, a large glass measuring cup, vegetable glycerin, distilled water, and a label.

Combine equal amounts of the herbs and weigh out 1½ ounces of the formula (save the rest for an infusion if you have extra) and pour it into the quart jar (this should fill about three-quarters of the jar). In a glass measuring cup, fill 240 milliliters vegetable glycerin and 160 milliliters distilled water. This will give you 60 percent vegetable glycerin out of 400 milliliters liquid. Mix this well until it is clear. Pour the liquid into the jar to the top slowly. Cap and label. Shake this daily and macerate for 4 weeks. Strain (I strain mine with a cheesecloth layered over a strainer sitting on top of a 4-cup measuring glass, then I gather the herb in cheesecloth and squeeze out the excess) and store in a cool and dark area.

🌿 *Fantastic! You made another remedy for the apothecary that everyone will enjoy!*

Goldenrod (*Solidago* spp.)

Taste: Pungent, slightly bitter, yet sweet
Qualities: Warming and drying
Parts used: Flowers and leaves
Medicinal properties: Alterative, antiphlogistic, antiseptic, astringent, carminative, digestive, diuretic, stimulant

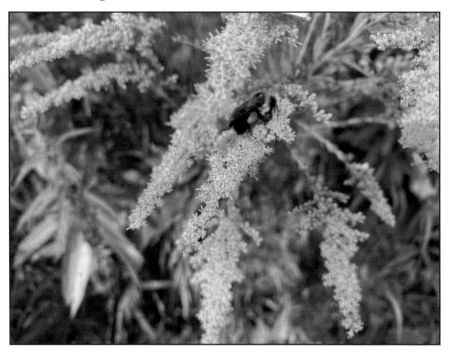

© Denise Cusack

Goldenrod species are easily noticed with their bright yellow flowers on tall stems waving in the wind in the fall season. They are often blamed for hay fever, but the pollen on this plant is only released by insects, whereas ragweed (*Ambrosia* spp.) growing nearby releases its pollen easily with the slightest wind. Both the flowers and the leaves provide the medicinal properties mentioned above. There are many different species of goldenrod growing in North America, and all are interchangeable in their actions. I have noticed three different kinds on my property alone.

As soon as the bright yellow flowers open, harvest about one foot of the stem containing both the leaves and the flowers. Use the fresh leaves and flowers in a tincture and hang the rest to dry for later use making infusions, other herbal preparations, or blends. You can infuse oil using the dried herb or make a poultice with the fresh herb topically for wounds due to the potent astringent and antiseptic properties. This is another herb that works well in standard dosing.

I usually can't wait to harvest this herb every fall. I rather enjoy sitting down to a nice warm infusion of goldenrod to help with some of my fall allergy symptoms. I will recommend this herb in a tincture or infusion for the start of any urinary tract infections, or to reduce the inflammation in the digestive tract. I feel this herb has an affinity not only for the kidneys and upper respiratory, but for the lungs as well. It can be useful in pulmonary and upper respiratory congestion to help thin the mucus and reduce the inflammation. I use it both as a simple (by itself) and in formulas when I make herbal preparations with it.

Exercise

Take the time in this exercise to make another warm infusion using the dried flowers and leaves of goldenrod. Cover and steep the herb for twenty minutes before straining. Document your personal take on the taste, actions, and energetics in your journal.

If you have the fresh herb available now, make a tincture using the folk method.

You will need: Fresh goldenrod flowers and leaves, 190 proof grain alcohol or 100 proof vodka, mason jar with lid, distilled water, label, and a bottle for storage

When using fresh flowers to make a tincture, pack the jar full of the herb. It is common knowledge that a higher alcohol content is needed with fresh flowers because of the extra water content in them; however, I have used 100 proof vodka as well when making a tincture, and I haven't noticed much of a difference in the medicinal actions. Choose either the grain alcohol or the vodka (or make two separate tinctures using both and compare the results). Once you pack the herb in the jar, either fill the jar ¾ of the way with the grain alcohol and the rest with the distilled water or fill it all the way to the top with the vodka. Cap and label the jar. Macerate for four weeks, then strain.

🌿 *Yet another herb or tincture ready for use in your apothecary.*

Ground Ivy (*Glechoma hederacea*)

Taste: Bitter and slightly acrid

Qualities: Warming and drying

Parts used: Herb (aerial parts)

Medicinal properties: Alterative, antioxidant, antiphlogistic, antispasmodic, astringent, carminative, cholagogue, digestive, diuretic, hepatic, nervine, pectoral, sialagogue, stimulant, tonic

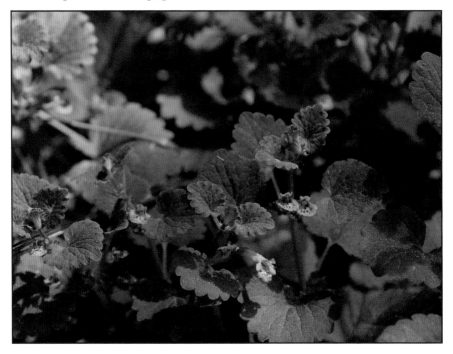

© Denise Cusack

Ground ivy goes by many different common names and is often thought of as an invasive weed in the yard. This is another springtime herb that offers a good amount of vitamin C in the leaves. The aerial parts of the plant are harvested and extracted for all the medicinal properties mentioned above. The best time to harvest will always be when the flowers first open, but you can harvest up until the hot weather of summer begins.

I collect the herb as soon as I can when the flowers open to make a fresh tincture, and then the rest is dried for use throughout the rest of the year. I prefer the infusion myself but will often recommend the tincture for my clients for convenience. Most of the time, I combine ground ivy with other herbs into a formula. I will also add the herb to my salads and smoothies for nutritional value. I use both drop and standard doses with this herb depending on the individual's need.

I feel this herb works great at thinning mucus and helping to reduce inflammation, and therefore, it would be a good choice for upper respiratory congestion in the sinus cavities and the ear. I include this herb along with immune modulators to help someone with sinusitis. I have heard other herbalists use it for tinnitus, but I have only found it to work some of the time depending on the cause since this condition can have different underlying causes. This is a good example of why we do not recommend herbs based on disease or symptoms alone, but rather the person and the cause. Ground ivy is also from the mint family and will act as an antispasmodic, carminative, and digestive herb for any stomach or intestinal issues such as IBS, stomach tension and cramping, flatulence, or slow and cold digestion. I also find this to be a stimulating alterative to move eliminatory channels when they have slowed down.

Exercise

For this exercise, I would like for you to take the time to taste an infusion made from both the fresh herb and the dried. Document the taste and actions of each on your body in your journal. Did you notice any changes? Do you prefer one over the other?

You can also prepare a fresh tincture using the same directions from the last exercise.

Compare the taste and actions from all three herbal preparations. When would you choose the tincture over the infusion? Would you recommend one over the other?

What part(s) of the body do you feel that this herb has an affinity for?

Research this herb and find other herbal preparations you can make with it. Would you use a different herbal preparation? Why?

Go back to all the previous herbs and make different preparations from them based on your research. Ask yourself the same questions and document your answers. You can continue this process with every herb in this chapter as you move forward.

Another tincture to add to your collection!

Hawthorn (*Crataegus* spp.)

Taste: Sweet and somewhat sour (berries), sour

Qualities: Cooling and moist (berries), cooling and drying (flowers and leaves)

Parts used: Berry, flower, and leaf

Medicinal properties: Antioxidant, antiphlogistic, astringent, cardiac tonic, digestive, diuretic, hypotensive

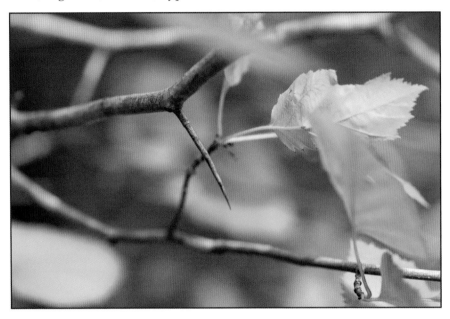

There are multiple Crataegus species in North America easily identified with the thorns, and each one is interchangeable in medicinal activity. Hawthorn berries are widely known to be a heart medicine tonic, and science is finding out the leaves also produce some of the same heart benefits while also confirming that the berries, leaves, and flowers are phytochemically similar in composition, differing in the ratios of a couple constituents.[21] Traditionally, hawthorn was also used for antioxidant, astringent, and diuretic purposes.

I collect the flowers and leaves in the spring to make a fresh tincture and fresh glycerite, and then I dry the rest for later use in infusions. The berries are collected in the fall, but I am having a hard time on this land finding berries that are free of blemishes as a result of pests or disease.

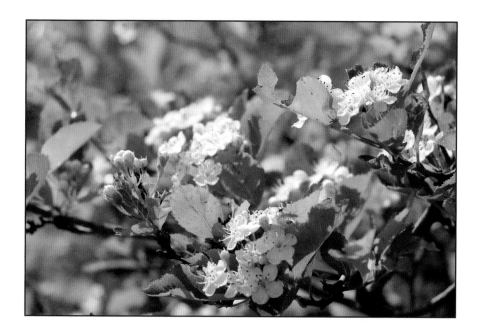

Because of this, I have been purchasing hawthorn berries, but I am also working more with the flowers and the leaves in my practice in place of the berries. I make the glycerite for children and for the adults that cannot have alcohol. Either that or I have them partake of this herb in an infusion. I will make a tincture using the dried hawthorn berries instead of the syrup to avoid the excess sugar content and when the fresh leaves or flowers are not available. I also make a flower essence with the flowers in the spring. Dosing for this herb is standard to maximum.

Hawthorn is considered a cooling astringent and is great for cooling heat and inflammation in the body. This is my go-to herb that I use for the circulatory system and the heart for its cardioprotective and trophorestorative actions. Hawthorn is a good choice to support the circulatory system in instances where there are palpitations, myocardial weakness, high/low blood pressure, high cholesterol, arrhythmia, or other heart diseases. I have also utilized hawthorn in cases where my clients suffer from edema, or they need support in clearing heat from the digestive system.

Exercise

For this exercise, I will let you decide which herbal preparation you want to make with this herb, and whether you want to use fresh, dried, or both.

Keep a detailed journal on your experiences.

Additionally, you can either grow seeds or plant the herb in a pot for your own garden. Research its germination requirements and growing conditions.

🌿 *Another herbal remedy at your disposal!*

Lemon Balm (*Melissa officinalis*)

Taste: Sour
Qualities: Cooling and drying
Parts used: Leaves
Medicinal properties: Antimicrobial, antioxidant, antispasmodic, anxiolytic, astringent, carminative, digestive, febrifuge, nervine, sedative

I named my first daughter Melissa and noticed that her name meant "bee." I had no idea why until I heard an old wives' tale say that lemon balm is to be rubbed on a beehive to bring bees home. This herb attracts bees in the garden, and upon further investigation, found out there is a deeper connection with the name Melissa and bees. The title Melissa, the bee, is a very ancient one; it constantly appears in Greek myths, sometimes belonging to a priestess or a nymph. One of the descriptors of Zeus was Melissaios, the "bee man." It is said he had a son by a nymph who, afraid of Hera's wrath, had the babe placed in a wood, where he was fed by bees. That nymph found the child and gave him the name Meliteus.[22] The leaves of this herb are used to create all of the above medicinal properties.

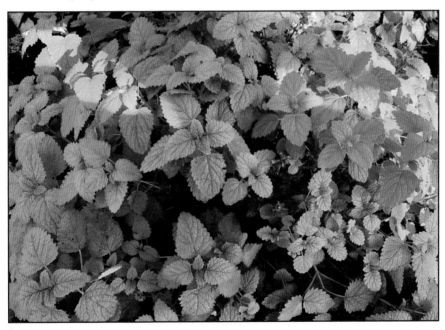

© Denise Cusack

I personally grow lemon balm in pots in my vegetable garden. As I stated earlier, this plant attracts bees, which will also help in pollinating my vegetables. I do not recommend growing this plant directly in the garden since it can be very invasive through the root system. As a matter of fact, harvest the leaves before flowering, and trim any flowers that open before they go to seed; otherwise, you will find them germinating where you do not want them. I like to collect the fresh leaves to make a tincture with and dry the rest for later use. I also combine this herb with other herbs in formulas using either water, alcohol, or glycerite as the menstruum. Most often, I use and recommend just the leaves in a warm infusion. Many people suggest fresh leaves are best, but I have found the dried leaves to be just as effective. Doses are standard.

I enjoy using lemon balm for its relaxing nervine and sedative actions on the body, and I will often enjoy a cup of warm infusion with this herb before bedtime. This is an herb I would suggest for children to calm them and help them relax in cases of ADHD, especially combined with adaptogens. I have also recommended this herb both internally and externally in shingles or other herpes outbreaks for its antiviral capabilities specific to this virus. It is helpful in digestive complaints, anxiety, tension headaches, insomnia, and hyperthyroidism. Studies have also shown an antitumor effect preventing the replication of cancer cells.[23]

Exercise

In this exercise, you will be making a hawthorn berry syrup.

You will need: 1 cup dried hawthorn berries, 4 cups distilled water, honey, and brandy (optional for preservation).

Start by soaking the dried berries in the distilled water overnight and adding a little more distilled water if needed to cover 2 inches above the berries. Place all in a saucepan (partially covered), bring to a boil, then reduce the heat to simmer and simmer until the liquid is reduced by half. Take off the heat, cover the pan, and let the liquid and herb steep for 20 minutes.

Strain, then add honey in a ratio of 2:1 with 2 parts decoction to 1 part honey. If desired for longer shelf life, add 25 percent brandy. Basically, ¼ cup brandy for every 1 cup decoction. Store syrup without the brandy in the refrigerator for 3 months. Syrup with brandy added can be stored for up to a year in the refrigerator.

🌿 Another herbal remedy at your disposal!

Linden (*Tilia* sp.)

Taste: Sweet

Qualities: Cooling and moistening

Parts used: Flowers and bracts and leaves

Medicinal properties: Antispasmodic, anxiolytic, demulcent, diaphoretic, diuretic, expectorant, nervine, sedative

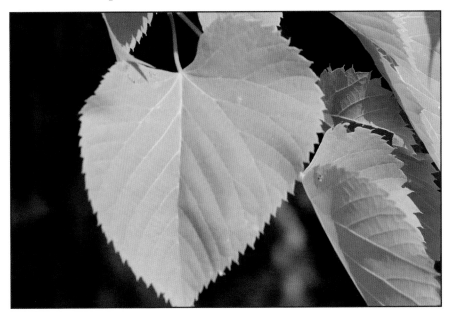

When I first moved into our previous home, I had a landscaping company come over and do some work for us. There was a tree I wasn't sure of and I asked the gentleman for its identification (this was before I became an herbalist). He told me it was a "weed tree" because he wasn't sure of its identification. That tree was American basswood (*Tilia americana*), or sometimes called American linden, and that tree became my focus to learn more about that species. The flowers and bracts produce all of the medicinal properties above, but the leaves have more mucilage content and therefore have more demulcent and expectorant properties.

I have found a tree at my current home too, and I collect the flowers and bracts in the early summer as they open to dry for use in my herbal preparations. I will also harvest the leaves throughout the growing season for fresh use as a poultice, and dried for baths and infusions. The dried flowers and bracts are used in infusions, baths, oils and ointments, tinctures, and fomentations. My first preference will always be the warm infusion for its comforting, soothing, and tasty qualities. Drop dosing and standard dosing are usually used with this herb, but you can use a maximum dosing for a shorter period of time.

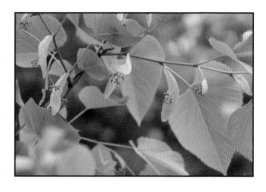

I will reach for linden to soothe my nerves, gladden my heart, relax my tension, and comfort my soul. It has a special connection to the emotional heart that doubles as a relaxing nervine that is gentle enough for everyone including children and the elderly. I use Linden similarly as lemon balm for children with ADHD, or those that need to slow down and relax. I choose which one to use based on the energetics of each individual. Where lemon balm is cooling and drying, Linden is cooling and moistening. I sometimes recommend Linden when a client of mine is suffering from grief. This can be from any type of loss. There's nothing like adding linden to a bath blend for soaking to soothe a tired mind and body.

Exercise

In this exercise, I want you to make a warm infusion with linden flowers and bracts one evening, then with lemon balm leaves another evening.

You will be experiencing two different sedative infusions of herbs at the same time one hour before bedtime (one infusion per night). Document smell, taste, actions, timing on effects, and any other feelings you might have with each.

Compare your findings. What did you learn?

🍃 Linden flowers and bracts add a special medicine to your apothecary whenever they are needed!

Marshmallow (*Althaea officinalis*)

Taste: Sweet and slightly salty
Qualities: Cooling and moistening
Parts used: Flowers, leaves, and root
Medicinal properties: Alterative, antiphlogistic, cell proliferant, demulcent, diuretic, emollient, expectorant, immunomodulant, nutritive, vulnerary

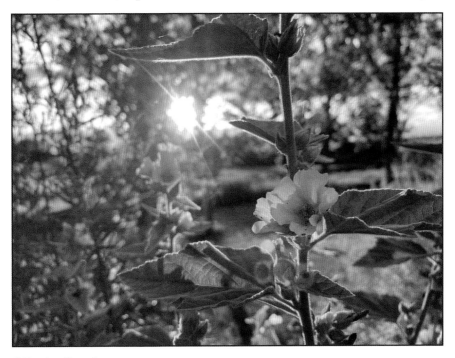

© Denise Cusack

This was one of the first herbs that I learned about when I began studying herbalism. I started to grow this herb immediately from seed and fell in love with both its beauty and medicinal properties. This is not the confection we all know, but the confection was probably named after it because the root was cooked, and the white pith scraped away as a sweet treat to enjoy. All parts of this herb will provide the same medicinal properties mentioned above. I think the root contains the most mucilage content of the three different parts, and it provides more of a demulcent, cell proliferant, and expectorant quality internally than the leaf and flower. However, the leaf and flower do contain mucilage and can be used as well.

During the growing season, I harvest the flowers as soon as they open to include in my salads for their nutritional value. The leaves are harvested throughout the growing season but have more mucilage content just before flowering. I cut the leaves up and dry them completely for later use in infusions, baths, or fomentations. You can use the leaves fresh as a poultice too. The root is dug in the fall from the second year or older plant and used either fresh or dried in a low alcohol tincture, a decoction, or cold infusion. Doses usually follow the standard philosophy.

I love marshmallow as a cell proliferant to repair the mucosal lining of the digestive tract, heal ulcers, and to speed the healing of internal or external tissue. It also makes a soothing and healing poultice for mastitis. I use it to help balance the immune system in cases of autoimmunity, and when a cooling and moistening herb is needed for heated and inflamed tissue especially in the lungs, kidneys, and digestive tract. Dr. Christopher even stated, "For obstinate inflammation and threatened mortification (gangrene), apply a poultice of the powdered or fresh crushed roots on the affected area as hot as possible and renew it before it dries." I find it especially beneficial for those suffering from a lingering cough, bronchitis, or asthma.

Exercise

You will be making a cold infusion using dried marshmallow root.

You will need: 2 tablespoons dried marshmallow root, ½ cup cold distilled water, a coffee grinder or small food processer, and pint jar with a cap.

Briefly pulse the dried root. Place the root in the jar and pour the measured cold water into the jar. Cap it, shake, and leave on the counter overnight. In the morning, strain the root out of the liquid and store the liquid in the refrigerator for use during the rest of the day. I recommend 2 tablespoons 3 times a day about an hour apart from any medications or food intake to soothe and repair. Higher dosages can be used for its expectorant properties if needed. You can also use this cold infusion externally for any rash, dry skin, or itchy conditions.

🌿 A popular herb to add to your apothecary!

Motherwort (*Leonurus cardiaca*)

Taste: Bitter

Qualities: Neutral and drying

Parts used: Herb

Medicinal properties: Antispasmodic, anxiolytic, cholagogue, diaphoretic, diuretic, emmenagogue, hepatic, nervine, sialagogue, tonic

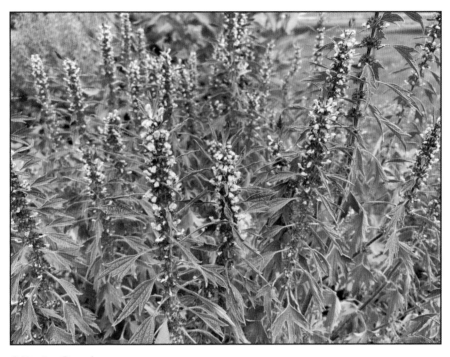

© Denise Cusack

I feel a special connection to motherwort. I actually dreamed about it and in my dream, I was harvesting this herb across the street. The dream reminded me to harvest it and when I woke up, I went across the street and did just that. A few hours later, all of the property across the street was mowed. If I didn't have that dream, I would have missed the opportunity to learn from this plant. What I have learned was that this is an extremely bitter plant that stimulated my liver while it helped to reduce my anxiety and regulate my cycle. I needed all of this at that time. Since then, motherwort has been one of my favorite plant allies. The entire herb is used in herbal medicine and produces all of the medicinal properties I provided above.

I harvest the top 4 to 6 inches of the plant as soon as the flowers open, and I immediately tincture the fresh herb. I will also dry what I have left to make a syrup, glycerite, fomentation, or an infusion when needed. If I need the bitter taste, I will use it as a tincture or infusion (not the easiest to get down due to the taste). If I am looking for the tonic properties for both the heart and uterus, or the nervine and antispasmodic properties, I will use the syrup or glycerite to sweeten it a bit for consumption. It can also be combined with sweet herbs if needed in a formula, but keep in mind what action you need first. This herb uses drop to standard doses medicinally.

For those with a uterus, motherwort is a constant companion through puberty, childbirth, premenopausal, and perimenopausal stages. I will use this for nervous afflictions caused by stress which can affect the heart, and for hormonal fluctuations. This is considered a cardiac and uterine tonic, but it can also help to balance the menstrual cycle in cases of amenorrhea and relieve spasms with dysmenorrhea. It can also be beneficial for acne prone skin caused by hormonal fluctuations. Postpartum depression, PMS, and hot flashes are other conditions that I look to supplement with motherwort if it is the right herb to balance the individual.

Exercise

This would be a good time to compare two different herbal preparations and their actions using fresh motherwort (dried if you don't have the fresh available). Be careful harvesting around the flowers because they do tend to prick the fingers. You will be making both a tincture and a syrup to compare.

You will need: Mason jar with lid, fresh or dried motherwort herb, 100 proof vodka, labels, distilled water, raw honey.

Pack the mason jar with the fresh herb or fill the jar halfway with the dried herb. Pour the vodka to the top of the jar and cap it. Label, shake it daily for 4 weeks, then strain it.

Make an infusion with either the fresh or dried herb. Let the herb steep in the distilled water, covered, for 20 minutes. Strain and add honey at ½ the volume or a 2:1 ratio of infusion to honey.

Document comparisons of actions, body parts affected, and taste in your journal. What were the differences?

🌿 *Two more remedies for the apothecary!*

Mullein (*Verbascum thapsus*)

Taste: Somewhat bitter and salty

Qualities: Cooling and moistening-neutral

Parts used: Flowers, leaves, and root

Medicinal properties: Analgesic, anodyne, anthelmintic, antimicrobial, antiphlogistic, antispasmodic, astringent, demulcent, diuretic, emollient, expectorant, lymphatic, vulnerary

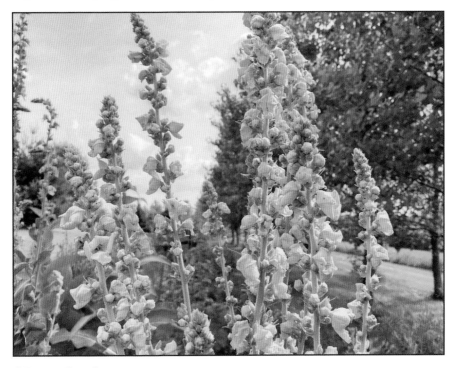

© Denise Cusack

This is another one of those beginner herbs for me, and one of the most used herbs in my formulas. There is such a wide array of uses and properties with mullein, and I find myself drawn to it often. Mullein is one of the "cure-all" herbs that works on multiple body systems. The integumentary (skin), lymph, respiratory, digestive, nervous, and musculoskeletal systems all can benefit from this herb. From my own personal experience, I believe that the different parts of this plant share some of the same medicinal properties. I know that there are some herbalists that say only the flowers can make an ear oil, or only the flowers can work on

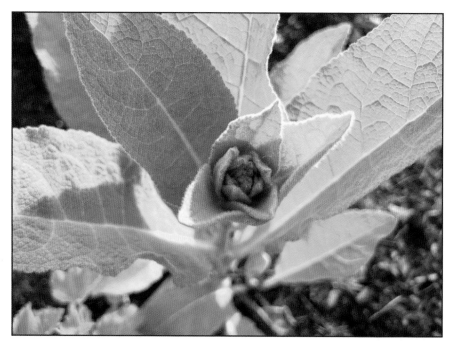
© Denise Cusack

the lymph, but I have tried many different applications using the different parts only to find that they seem interchangeable.

Mullein is a biennial plant that grows the leaves the first year, and the flowers and stalk the second year. After that, the plant releases the seed and dies. With this in mind, I like to harvest the leaves from the first-year plant, the root from the first-year plant, and the flowers as soon as they open in the second year. I use fresh or dried flowers and leaves for use in infusions, low-alcohol tinctures, fomentations, oils, or ointments. The roots are harvested and used to make a low-alcohol tincture, decoction, oil, or ointment. The leaves are covered in irritating little hairs, and they should be strained twice using a cheesecloth or coffee filter to capture all of the tiny hairs before consumption. Standard dosing applies.

As I mentioned, I use mullein in many of my formulas to relieve inflammation and pain, and break up congestion in the lungs, ears, and lymph system. I also use it to help expectorate mucus from the lungs, reduce glandular swelling, reduce swelling in the joints, and help soothe nerve pain and discomfort. I like to include mullein in formulas with other herbs to help direct where it goes in the body, support its medicinal properties, and for added support to all those different body systems. I include it in ointments for external use because it is antimicrobial, antispasmodic, anodyne, lymphatic, vulnerary, nervine, and antiphlogistic properties. It really covers many of the actions needed for external applications.

Exercise

Since I mentioned that I have seen the flowers, leaves, and roots provide some of the same medicinal properties, I want you to make herbal preparations of each to compare for yourself. You can choose the same menstruum to extract each part. If you choose water, you will make an infusion of both the leaves and flowers, and a decoction for the roots. If you choose alcohol, use a 25 percent alcohol content (I use 195 proof Everclear and only fill ¼ of the jar using dried materials and the rest with distilled water). You can infuse separate oils with each part too.

This exercise could take some time for you to document your findings in your journal, have different people try it, and experiment with different afflictions. Take your time with this experiment. Document everybody's results to gain better insight.

🌿 *You just added multiple preparations containing one herb to your apothecary!*

Nettle (*Urtica dioica*)

Taste: Sweet and salty
Qualities: Considered neutral
Parts used: Herb, root, seeds
Medicinal properties: Alterative, antihistamine, antioxidant, antiphlogistic, diuretic, nutritive, rubefacient, tonic, trophorestorative

Almost every herbalist joyfully celebrates when they see a patch of nettles growing near them. It is common knowledge that this plant offers multiple medicinal benefits and is restorative to the entire body. Nettle is often called, "stinging nettle" due to the hairs on the edge of the leaves that inject a compound of chemicals into the animal or person that brushes up against it. It is this compound that creates the lasting sting. This sting has been used in the past to reduce pain and inflammation. It is called *urtication*. Fortunately, other compounds contribute to the antiphlogistic benefits when taken internally too. All parts of this herb can be used medicinally, although each herbalist has their favorite part for certain actions in the body. Some like the seeds as a tonic for the

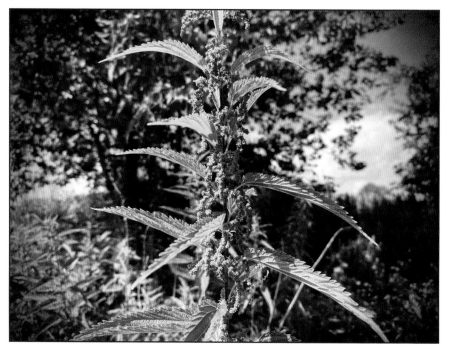

© Denise Cusack

endocrine system, but I find the leaves and root work the same. As you gain experience with this herb, you can come to your own conclusion as to which part to use for the properties above.

I harvest the young leaves in the spring before they flower by cutting the top four inches of the plant, or at least the first few pairs of leaves. Grab the top and bottom of the leaf or wear gloves to avoid getting stung by the hairs on the edge. I will include them in my cooking and baking or make a fresh tincture, then save the rest to dry for later use during the year. I used to gather the seeds after flowering but now prefer to just use the herb itself in my practice. I gather the roots in the fall. I like to make a warm infusion using nettle leaves 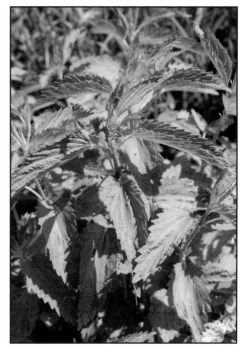 combined with other herbs in a formula. For convenience, the fresh tincture can also be combined with other tinctured herbs in a formula or used alone as a simple. This herb is often recommended in standard to maximum doses.

I use this herb when my clients are weakened either by certain health conditions, outside factors, or nutritional deficiencies. I also like to use it to relieve inflammation, stimulate the kidneys, and as an anti-allergenic. It restores function in all systems of the body and acts as a strengthener. I have used nettle as a hair rinse to strengthen the follicles and restore sebaceous gland function in cases of hair loss and dry scalp conditions. I would also use the herb internally for both in addition to the hair rinse. I love combining nettle with rose petals in a warm infusion. It is one of my favorites.

Exercise

If you have the plant nearby to harvest from, look up different recipes using the fresh herb and try them at home.

Use the dried leaves to make 4 cups of a warm infusion. You can use either a pan or a large teapot to infuse the leaves. Let this cool a bit and use this as a hair rinse after you shampoo, but don't rinse it out. Document your results and experience in your journal after using this for the next week (make a new infusion each time).

You can also leave some or make another cup of the warm infusion for drinking. Try drinking the standard dose for a week. Document your results, the energetics, and the taste in your journal.

🍃 A great multiuse herb for your apothecary!

Oats (*Avena sativa*)

Taste: Sweet

Qualities: Cooling and moistening

Parts used: Milky seed tops, straw (dried stems)

Medicinal properties: Antispasmodic, demulcent, emollient, nervine, nutritive, tonic, trophorestorative, vulnerary

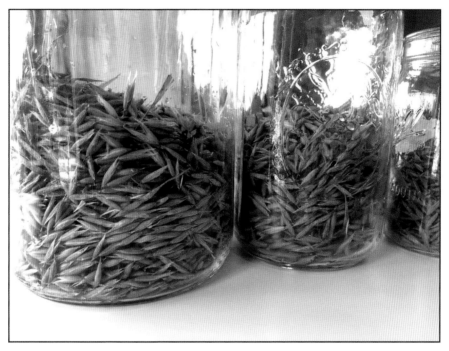

© Denise Cusack

This grain has been a staple as both a food and medicine for thousands of years. The seeds can either be used in the milky stage for medicine or dried as mature seeds for food. The milky seed tops are harvested when you gently squeeze the seeds and see white latex escaping. These seeds are generally preferred as a nervine tonic, trophorestorative, cardiac tonic, and antispasmodic. Oatstraw and oatmeal are both considered nutritive, demulcent, emollient, and vulnerary. The nutritional value of oats could also be partly responsible for the tonic and trophorestorative properties.

I like to use the oat plant as a cover crop for my gardens. This gives me access to the medicine, and my soil continues to reap the benefits once they are turned under. I plant the seed as soon as the soil is ready around the time that I plant my peas. The seeds are in the milky stage after flowering and before the heat of the summer, which are harvested and made into a fresh tincture or glycerite. The extra seed that I harvested can be dried along with some of the stems that I collected at the same time for use in a warm infusion, bath, ointment, or fomentation when they are needed throughout the rest of the year. You can enjoy a bath for the soothing emollient properties. Since this herb is a tonic, either standard doses over a longer period of time, or larger doses can be used medicinally.

I consider oats a long-term restorative to the nervous, endocrine, and cardiovascular system. I will choose to add oats for a client who has had long-term effects of trauma, a hormone imbalance, chronic stress related symptoms, or is currently suffering from addiction and needs additional nerve support. I like to combine oats with other nervines, adaptogens, cardiovascular tonics, and demulcents in formulas for my clients.

Exercise

Take the time in the next growing season to harvest your own milky oat tops to make a fresh tincture. You will pack a Mason jar full and pour ¾ of the jar full of Everclear 195 proof. Fill the rest of the jar with distilled water, put the lid on, label, and shake daily for one month.

Alternatively, purchase oatstraw from a reputable source or dry your own milky oat tops and stems to make a warm infusion. Compare the properties of both a fresh tincture of the milky sap and the oatstraw in a warm infusion and document these in your journal. (You can purchase a tincture of the fresh milky oat tops if you do not have the opportunity to harvest them yourself.)

🍃 A special nerve tonic just added to your apothecary!

Peppermint (*Mentha piperita*)

Taste: Pungent

Qualities: Warming at first and drying with a cool aftereffect

Parts used: Herb

Medicinal properties: Analgesic, antimicrobial, antiphlogistic, antispasmodic, anodyne, carminative, diaphoretic, digestive, emmenagogue, febrifuge, nervine, rubefacient, stimulant, stomachic

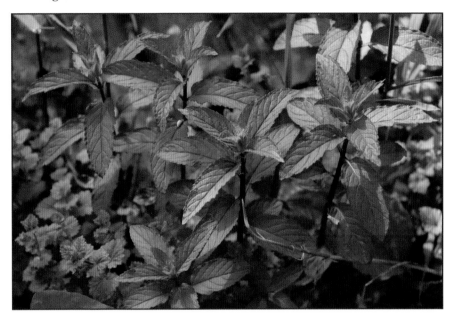

Most people are familiar with this plant, its taste, and its ability to aid digestion and alleviate nausea. It is commonly found as a simple in the grocery store aisle amongst the tea varieties. It is also a captivating aromatic herb that stimulates the senses. The entire herb can be utilized for all of the medicinal properties mentioned above. If the aroma is sought for medicinal applications, the leaves can be crushed and the scent inhaled, or the essential oil can be used for longer lasting scent and convenience. A variety called chocolate mint is a delicious alternative.

As for growing any of the mints, it is best to have them in separate pots rather than in the ground. They spread by underground runners, and they will take over your gardens and smother some of the other plants. I learned this the hard way, and I also learned not to plant peppermint with spearmint. Spearmint will eventually overtake peppermint in due time! I will also not grow them in a raised bed because their roots grow below the soil, through the cloth barrier, and into the yard. So, pots it is! I like to cut the stems as they grow to use fresh in my herbal preparations and for beverages. This little bit of cutting throughout the season will stimulate more growth. I will use the rest throughout the season to air dry in a well-ventilated room out of direct sunlight for later use. I will use them in ointments, oils, infusions, baths, and fomentations. I like using peppermint as a simple and in formulas with other herbs. Doses are drop dosing to standard dosing.

Peppermint is a pungent herb that is also a digestive. Both of these combined are the reasons why I will often utilize this to disperse mucus in the digestive tract, stimulate the digestive process, and stimulate the appetite. Its initial warming energetic will also act to move its medicinal properties quickly throughout the body while its cooling aftereffects will help reduce heat in the digestive system and soothe inflammatory tissue. I use peppermint externally for spasms, pain associated with inflammation, or pain associated with the nerves. When someone suffers from a fever and also has nasal congestion, I recommend a hot cup of the infusion to sip on while inhaling the steam.

Exercise

In this exercise, you will infuse olive oil with peppermint leaves for external use.

You will need: Double boiler, 8 ounces organic olive oil, 7 grams peppermint leaves, cheesecloth, strainer, large glass measuring cup, dark bottle, and label.

Add water to the bottom of your double boiler and the olive oil and herb to the top pan. Bring the water to a gentle boil and simmer (covered) for one hour, stirring occasionally. Place the cheesecloth over the strainer and place the strainer on a large glass measuring cup. Pour the infused oil into the cheesecloth and strainer and let the oil drain. Once the oil is cooled, pour into a dark bottle and label it.

🌿 *A great base for other remedies just added to your apothecary!*

Plantain (*Plantago* spp.)

Taste: Slightly bitter
Qualities: Cooling and moistening with some drying aspects
Parts used: Leaves, root, and seeds
Medicinal properties: Alterative, anodyne, antiphlogistic, antimicrobial, antioxidant, astringent, cell proliferant, demulcent, depurant, diuretic, emollient, expectorant, hemostatic, hepatic, hepatoprotective, lymphatic, vulnerary

Plantain is one of the first herbs that most herbalists learn namely due to its many uses and its availability. It might be thought of as a common weed, but it is a powerhouse of an herb. Dr. Christopher referred to it as, "The best herb for blood poisoning." Two of the most common are *Plantago lanceolata* and *P. major*, but where I live, we have a native *P. rugelii* that I use. The leaves are harvested for all of the medicinal actions mentioned above. The leaves and roots have specific alterative effects on the circulatory

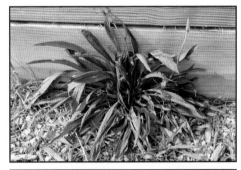
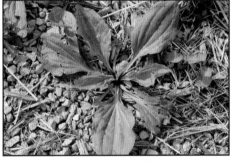

and lymph system. The seeds sold commercially are called psyllium and are harvested from *P. psyllium* or *P. ovata*. You can collect the seeds from our local species as well, or just utilize the leaves. I harvest the leaves before flowering for the most potency to make a fresh tincture and to dry for future use in an ointment or infusion, but I will also harvest them fresh throughout the growing season when needed, or when my supply is getting lower. A warm infusion can be taken internally, added to bath water, or be used with a fomentation when moist heat is preferred externally. Standard to maximum dosage is used with this herb.

Living in a rural area, I often reach for plantain leaves as a poultice for bug bites, insect stings, poison ivy, cuts, or infected cuts. The astringency in plantain has a drawing effect to draw out venom, saliva from mosquitos, stingers, or infections. It also soothes irritated, swollen, or painful tissue due to rashes, insects, or other plants. I will use it internally in cases where poison ivy is spreading quickly in an individual, and I need to move it out of their system. This will help to eliminate the spreading and lasting effects of the rash. It is also beneficial for systemic inflammation, chronic infections, and pulmonary issues. As a diuretic with soothing mucilage, it helps to reduce kidney inflammation and repair the cells. It also has reparative and protective properties in the liver.

Exercise

In this exercise, you will research which Plantago *species grows near you and find some. Once you find it, harvest some of the leaves to make a fresh warm infusion and dry the rest for later use. Document the taste of fresh versus dried plantain infusion.*

When a mosquito bites you or a bee stings you, grab some fresh leaves to use as a poultice. Chew the leaves and place them directly on the affected bite or sting until it dries. Reapply if needed. What happened to the symptoms? How long did it take? Document this experience in your journal.

🌿 Another top-notch first aid herb added to your inventory!

Raspberry (*Rubus idaeus*)

Taste: Sweet with a slight sour aftertaste

Qualities: Cooling and drying

Parts used: Leaves and fruit

Medicinal properties: Alterative, analgesic, antimicrobial, antioxidant, astringent, diuretic, emmenogogue, galactogogue, hemostatic, nutritive, stomachic, tonic

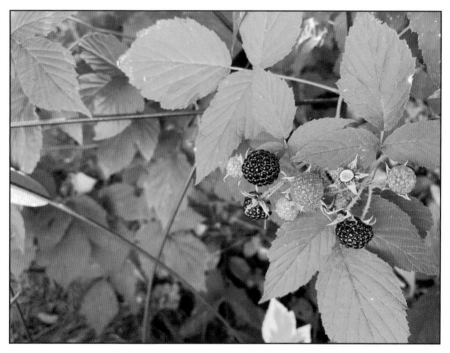

© Denise Cusack

Red raspberry canes are very invasive and are readily available throughout my area. Most are the wild variety (*R. strigosus* or *R. occidentalis*) instead of the cultivated *R. idaeus*. This is an herb that I have stocked in my medicine chest over the years simply because of the wide variety of uses, and the great taste which children will often consume without too much of a fight. Blackberries (*R. villosus*, *R. fruticosus*) were used more often in the past and can be used interchangeably. The sweet taste indicates a higher nutritive value, and the leaves show a manganese content twice that of other herbs with a very high niacin and iron content included.

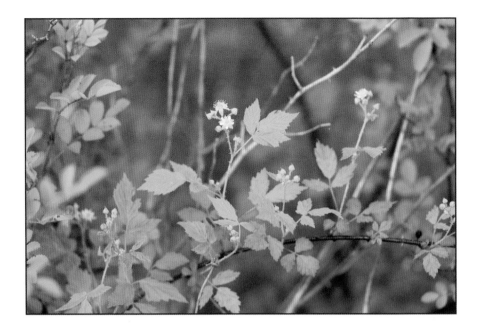

I collect the leaves in the spring before the flowering begins for the most potent medicinal activity, but I will harvest them all throughout the growing season when they are needed. I mostly use the dried leaves in warm infusions, fomentations, washes, or baths; however, I will make a fresh leaf tincture to have on hand to mix in a custom formula for my clients.

I use red raspberry leaves to alleviate diarrhea, sore throat, hemorrhoids, nausea, and vomiting. It is considered a very good astringent to tone and contract tissue which also helps in the leakage of excess fluid from the body. I was taught by the teachings of Dr. Christopher to use this as an eyewash in the prevention of macular degeneration and cataracts. With the hemostatic action, it can also help slow down the bleeding of retinopathy, menstruation, or hemorrhaging after childbirth. As an antioxidant containing large amounts of vitamin C, I also like to make a warm infusion at the beginning of any cold or flu to shorten the duration of each. This can be made as a warm infusion, but then cooled and used as iced tea if it is preferred. I mostly use it as a simple, but I will include it in some of my tea blends as an astringent, nutritive, and antioxidant. It is usually referred to as "the pregnancy herb" due to its ability as a uterine tonic, hemostatic, analgesic, anti-nausea, and galactagogue.

Exercise

For this exercise, I would like for you to collect the leaves or purchase them to make a warm infusion. Taste the warm infusion and document the taste along with the actions in your body.

Take that same infusion and use it as an external wash and a gargle. Document what happened.

Take that same infusion and proceed with an eyewash. Sterilize two eyecups (or shot glasses) and use only one glass per eye. Fill them halfway with the warm infusion, place the cup over the eye with your head bent forward, then tip your head back to let the fluid enter the eye. Place a towel below the cup to catch drippage. Do the same for the other eye with the next cup. How different does your eye feel?

🍃 *Multiple applications for this herb to be used in your apothecary!*

Red clover (*Trifolium pratense*)

Taste: Sweet

Qualities: Somewhat cooling but can benefit all different energetic qualities

Parts used: Flowers

Medicinal properties: Alterative, anticancer (antiproliferative: prohibiting cell growth and spread), antispasmodic, depurative, diuretic, emmenagogue, hepatic, lymphatic, nervine, nutritive

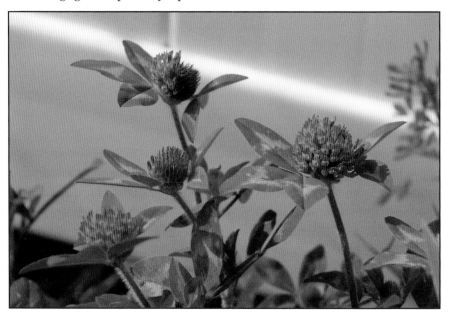

Red clover is considered a highly nutritious herb and is delicious to boot! It is taller than the common white clover (*T. repens*) with larger leaves and a reddish-purple flower. Being a legume, it is also used as a cover crop to add much-needed nitrogen to the soil. The flowering tops are the medicinal part of the herb that contributes to the medicinal properties.

As soon as the first blossoms start to appear and open, I will collect as many as I can to dry indoors out of the hot sun and humidity with good ventilation. If done right without excessive heat or humidity, the blossoms will retain the color and not turn brown. When the blossoms are picked more often, the plant will give more flower production. I do collect the blossoms throughout the growing season whenever they appear to make a fresh tincture and dry the rest for later use throughout the year. Standard to maximum dosage is used with this herb.

Red clover was the subject of my thesis in school. It was traditionally used internally for whooping cough based on the alterative and antispasmodic actions of this herb. It was also traditionally used as a skin wash to relieve inflammation with eczema and psoriasis. I once checked to see if it was safe for canines and made tea for my dog when she had kennel cough. She couldn't even bark prior to taking it without having a coughing fit. Immediately afterward, she stopped coughing, and it never came back. I use both the raw blossoms directly in my diet, or in a warm infusion for its nutritive benefits. I most often include red clover blossoms in different blends as a warm infusion or added to formulas as a tincture. I rarely use it as a simple, and I find that it combines well with other alteratives, hepatics, nervines, lymphatics, and antispasmodics. This herb works to balance the endocrine system and is used to help balance the hormones in all individuals. This includes hot flashes and night sweats, and benign prostatic hyperplasia (BPH). In my practice, this herb is a standard in formulas for my clients concerned with cancer either as a preventative, or in some active cases.

Exercise

For this exercise, I would like for you to collect the blossoms or purchase them to make a tincture. Combine the blossoms with 75 percent alcohol content and 25 percent distilled water using the folk method (pack the jar with fresh blossoms) and make a separate tincture using dried blossoms with 50 percent alcohol content and 50 percent water (fill the jar halfway with dried blossoms).

Take both tinctures internally after the four 4 of maceration and document to compare the different possible actions and strengths.

🌿 *More tinctures added!*

Rosemary (*Salvia rosmarinus*, previously known as *Rosmarinus officinalis*)

Taste: Pungent
Qualities: Warming and drying
Parts used: Herb
Medicinal properties: Anthelmintic, antifungal, antimicrobial, antioxidant, antispasmodic, astringent, carminative, digestive, diuretic, emmenagogue, nervine, rubefacient, stimulant

Rosemary is a common culinary herb, but it also has an extensive history medicinally. It is known as the "memory herb" since it was used traditionally to help refresh and stimulate the memory and cognitive thinking. This was done by carrying the sprigs, crushing them, and inhaling the fragrance. Rosemary has been utilized for centuries while being a staple in the garden of every home. Having this herb grow in the garden or stored in the cupboards is beneficial as a culinary spice, an herbal medicine, and as an aromatic. The aerial parts are 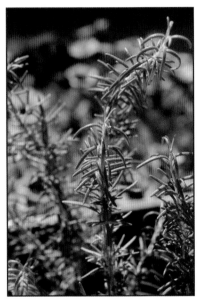 responsible for all of the medicinal properties mentioned.

I prefer to bring my plant indoors for the winter to keep enjoying the fresh herb in my cooking or to use medicinally all season long. Once the weather warms, I will put it back outside in my garden. I harvest the fresh leaves to be used for a warm infusion, a tincture, a glycerite, an infused vinegar, and infused oil or ointment, or for an infused honey. Sometimes, I will have a larger harvest and I will need to dry what I cannot use at the time. It is important to not use a heat source to dry this aromatic herb to preserve its potency as medicine. I just lay mine out on a screen indoors with a good airflow. I can use the dried herb the same way as I use the fresh, but I prefer to use fresh over dried.

As I am sitting here, I have a rolling applicator containing olive oil and rosemary essential oil that I put together as an aromatic and an external application to help stimulate my memory while I am writing. I roll this above my lips so that I can inhale the aroma without having to hold the essential oil under my nose. I also have a formula that includes both the herb and the essential oil along with other antispasmodic and anodyne herbs to help with tension, spasms, inflammation, and pain. I love making an infusion of the whole herb for use in a spray bottle, or to add to my bath. The spray bottle can be used as an antimicrobial for surfaces, as a leave-in conditioner for the hair and scalp, or as an insecticidal. I use rosemary in my practice as a stimulant of the circulatory system, a warming herb needed in my formulas, a nervine, an antispasmodic, a digestive antimicrobial, a hepatoprotective, or an antifungal. There are so many uses with this herb, and it can easily be combined with other herbs to complete a formula.

Exercise

You will be making an infused honey for this exercise.

You will need a jar packed with dried rosemary, raw unpasteurized local honey, and the sun. (Commercial rosemary is lacking many of the medicinal benefits since heat is often used to "sanitize" it. Compare coloring and aromatics of your dried herb with the commercially dried herb.)

Once the jar is packed with the herb, fill the jar with the honey. Cap this and label it. Place this jar in the full sun while rotating it daily by flipping the jar upside down for a day, then right side up the next day. Let the honey infuse for 1 month. At the end of this time, strain the honey and keep it in a jar in a cool and dark area.

🍃 *Another great herb and base added to your apothecary!*

Saint-John's-wort (*Hypericum perforatum*)

Taste: Sweet and slightly bitter

Qualities: Warming and drying

Parts used: Herb

Medicinal properties: Alterative, analgesic, anodyne, antimicrobial, antiphlogistic, antispasmodic, anxiolytic, astringent, cholagogue, digestive, diuretic, hepatic, nervine, vulnerary

Saint-John's-wort has a recent reputation as an alternative herb for antidepressants. This sunny herb can help with mild depression, but there is so much more to this plant. It was once called the blood of Christ because the infused oil turns red resembling the color of his blood as it performs healing attributions. The aerial parts are used in herbal preparations to provide all the medicinal properties mentioned above.

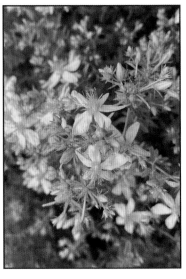

© Denise Cusack

I only take one third of each plant that I find in the wild by cutting the top four inches as soon as the flowers open. I immediately make a fresh tincture with these, and I will wilt some of the fresh flowers for just one day to solar infuse in an oil. Some herbalists say to use the fresh flowers only to infuse in the oil, but since oil and water don't mix, I prefer to wilt mine briefly before preparing it. You can also use the dried herb to infuse in an oil and get the same medicinal properties. I will also dry some of the herb for later use to make infusions. This herb uses all dosing measurements depending on the need.

This is one of the best herbs to take both internally and externally with shingles. It is an antiviral, a nervine relaxant, and it helps to reduce the pain tremendously in those cases. I also use this herb internally and externally for neuralgia, sciatica, or neuroma pain. I include this herb internally in formulas with seasonal affective disorder, feelings of anxiety, withdrawal symptoms, and melancholy. I have found Saint-John's-wort to be a valuable antispasmodic externally for those suffering from hyper-tonic pelvic dysfunction syndrome, restless leg syndrome, and fibromy-algia. One thing to know about this herb is the contraindications and interactions. It is usually not recommended with pharmaceutical medi-cations due to the ability to speed up the detoxification processes. So generally, if someone is on medications, I will not recommend this herb.

Exercise

It is a good idea for you to understand why the fresh herb of Saint-John's-wort is said to be preferred for use in herbalism, and if it is necessary. Determine the differ-ences and similarities of a solar-infused oil using the fresh herb in one jar and the dried herb in the other. You can also wilt the fresh herb for one day as an experiment.

With the fresh or wilted herb, pack a jar full and pour organic olive oil to fill the jar to the top. Poke the herb with a stick or spoon to let out some air pockets. Cap this, label it, and store outside in the sun for at least 2 weeks. For the dried herb, fill the jar halfway, then pour in the olive oil until it reaches the top of the jar.

Make sure all oils are macerated for the same length of time and preferably in the same spot to receive the same amount of sunlight. Document your findings and your preferences after using each.

🍃 *A popular first aid oil just added to the apothecary shelf!*

Self-heal (*Prunella vulgaris*)

Taste: Combination of slight bitter, sweet, and salty
Qualities: Cooling and moistening with a secondary drying action
Parts used: Herb as the flowers first open, or mature flowerheads
Medicinal properties: Alterative, antimicrobial, antiphlogistic, antispasmodic, astringent, cholagogue, demulcent, diuretic, emollient, expectorant, febrifuge, hepatic, lymphatic, stomachic, tonic, vulnerary

Self-heal is a versatile plant with many different applications in herbal medicine. It was once called heal-all based on the multiple healing properties of this herb. It works in an upward direction at first working on the sinus cavities and then moving downward through the lymph system and digestive track. I personally feel that self-heal could be considered "binding" with its astringent properties and mucilaginous content since it both binds and heals tissue. Interestingly enough, this herb has the inhibitory effects of preventing the binding of certain viruses by preventing entry to cells.[24]

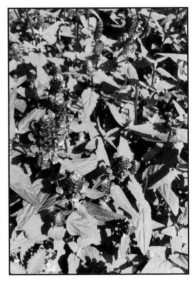

I usually find this herb flowering beginning in the early summer in my area. As with other herbs, frequent harvesting of the plant will give you more growth and opportunities for a later harvest. I cut the herb to include the flower, stem, and leaves, and I use this fresh or dried for my herbal preparations. I like to make a fresh tincture and dry the rest in a warm infusion, cold infusion, syrup, infused oil, or bath. The fresh herb also makes a healing poultice, drawing agent, or hemostatic in external applications. Standard dosing is utilized with this herb and sometimes larger doses being that it is considered a tonic.

I first and foremost like self-heal as a repairing and restorative agent to the respiratory and digestive system. I also find it a gentle lymph mover, a powerful antimicrobial, and a modulator of the immune system. It shares similar actions with plantain, but they are not completely similar. You will only know the difference by experimenting with them both yourself. I like to pick this herb in the woodland trails, or edge of the woods as a poultice for mosquito bites or other bug bites, to help a wound heal, or to relieve a rash when I cannot spot plantain in the vicinity. I often combine self-heal with other alteratives, demulcents, and emollients, or digestive herbs in a formula rather than as a simple herb alone.

Exercise

This is a great opportunity for you to take the time to compare tastes, energetics, and properties of both self-heal and plantain. Document these comparisons as different herbal preparations using both fresh and dried herbs.

Did you find a difference in taste, energetics, and their actions?

Did you find a difference in potency between the two herbs, or between using fresh or dried of each?

Would you stock both in your medicine chest, or one over the other? Why?

If you have an opportunity to try both with a health condition, try them and document your experience. An example would be with a cough. Which acts as a better expectorant? Do they work better together? This is the best way to gain experience and connect with each herb.

🌿 *Can't go wrong with adding heal-all to your apothecary!*

Skullcap (*Scutellaria lateriflora*)

Taste: Slightly bitter

Qualities: Cooling and drying

Parts used: Herb

Medicinal properties: Analgesic, antimicrobial, antioxidant, antispasmodic, anxiolytic, astringent, diaphoretic, diuretic, emmenagogue, nervine, sedative, tonic, trophorestorative

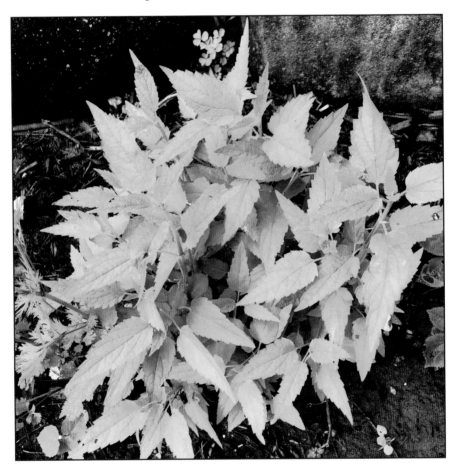

© Denise Cusack

Skullcap is a very well-known nerve tonic and trophorestorative. It rebuilds, tones, relaxes, and strengthens the entire nervous system. It was once called mad-dog skullcap due to its popularity in the past as a remedy for hydrophobia (a symptom of rabies) according to Mrs. M.

Grieve. Dr. Christopher refers to it as "one of the best nervine agents that nature provides." The aerial parts are harvested for all of the medicinal properties provided above.

I have harvested from both plantings in my garden, and from the wild. It will be easiest to buy the plants for direct planting in your gardens. I have found that wild skullcap is not easily found, nor does it always show up in the same place from year to year. I do know that if you plant them directly in your garden, you should keep them moist and in a partly shaded location where they do not get full sun all day long. I harvest the top one third of the plant to make a fresh tincture then dry more for later use. Dry this herb in a well-ventilated shaded area, and immediately transfer it to an airtight container. This herb usually follows standard dosing but can definitely be used in all dosing applications depending on the need. Larger doses have a sedative effect.

Suffice it to say, I include skullcap in almost all of my nerve formulas. I rely on this herb as a tonic for the nervous system, which can be taken for longer periods of time. This includes cases of withdrawal symptoms, anxiety, insomnia, stress, epileptic episodes, adult ADHD, and PMS. I most often use it in formulas rather than as a simple, except in cases of withdrawal. It is strong enough as a simple to affect the individual positively. I do not think of this herb as a strong diuretic or diaphoretic, and I will usually choose another herb with these properties. However, it does combine nicely with other herbs that are stronger, which can add to the effects. This herb is from the mint family, so I find it beneficial for nervous and tense stomachs and digestive cramping as well.

Exercise

For this exercise, I would like for you to compare the similarities and differences between skullcap tinctures (or warm infusions) made from fresh and dried herbs. Make these when you have the opportunity. (If you cannot find it in the wild, or grow it yourself, ask around to herbalists in your community for a resource.)

Document your findings in your journal.

🍃 *Another great herb or tincture to have on hand in the apothecary!*

Sweet leaf (*Monarda fistulosa*)

Taste: Pungent and slightly sweet

Qualities: Warming and drying

Parts used: Flowers and leaves

Medicinal properties: Alterative, antimicrobial, antispasmodic, astringent, carminative, diaphoretic, digestive, diuretic, emmenagogue, febrifuge, lymphatic, nervine, stimulant

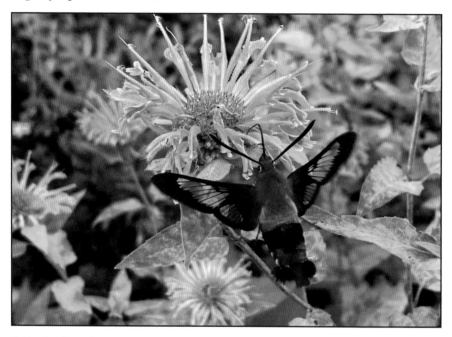

© Denise Cusack

I looked for this herb for many years before it literally came to me. I lived in the same home for over eleven years without a sighting, and all of a sudden it bloomed across the street one day. I also began planting it in my gardens. We moved into our new home that we built a few years later, and I was worried I wouldn't find any. I worried for nothing as there are large patches of sweet leaf throughout the woods on this property. It showed up in spades, and I don't need to grow it in my gardens! Needless to say, this is an herb I use often and for many of the medicinal properties documented above. The flowers are more pungent in flavor and therefore not as desired as the leaves, but I like to include both in my herbal preparations. Other common names are bee balm and wild bergamot.

Starting in the later spring, I will begin collecting the aromatic leaves before they start to have insect damage or powdery mildew. Once the blooms open, I collect the top six to eight inches of undamaged leaves and flowers. I include the fresh leaves and flowers to make a tincture while saving the rest for use in other herbal preparations. Throughout the season, I will collect more if I need to. I love sitting down to drink the warm infusion, which will give you a nice relaxing feeling and stimulate its diaphoretic property. I also add fresh or dried leaves to my cooking since it contains the same aromatics as oregano (*Origanum vulgare*) and is sometimes called wild oregano. Dosing used with this herb is usually drop or standard.

I like using sweet leaf for fevers to release the heat and when there is heat deep within the tissues. I love combining this herb with other nervines, antispasmodics, and digestives. In all instances where oregano is used in herbal medicine, I will often use sweet leaf instead since it is readily available in my area. I include it in my bone broths, fire cider, nervine blends, digestive blends, and bath blends. It makes a very relaxing and aromatic bath! I also find it a worthwhile alterative, stimulating the lymph, kidneys, and circulation.

Exercise

Harvest both the flowers and leaves when you have an opportunity to use them in a warm infusion. Try them individually, then together. Any difference in its taste and actions? Which plant part do you prefer? If you do not have access to the flowers, purchase the dried leaves to make a warm infusion.

Add the dried leaves to your cooking in place of oregano. Document in your journal the taste and actions on your body. How does this compare to other mints for you? Does it excel in other areas? Do you prefer oregano or sweet leaf in your cooking? Why?

🌿 *One of my favorite herbs just added to your apothecary!*

Teasel (*Dipsacus sylvestris*)

Taste: Bitter and pungent
Qualities: Warming and drying
Parts used: Root
Medicinal properties: Analgesic, antiphlogistic, antispasmodic, astringent, cholagogue, hemostatic, hepatic, stimulant

I didn't find a lot of information about teasel when I first began studying. I stumbled upon information in *The Earthwise Herbal* about the root being used for joint pain, and I have personally suffered from joint pain myself. I began my research on this herb and started taking it off and on for a few years. The medicinal properties I have for this herb are based on my own experience using the root in an alcoholic herbal preparation. Teasel has been used as a Yang tonic, bone healer, hemostatic, and antirheumatic. Specifically,

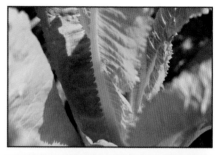

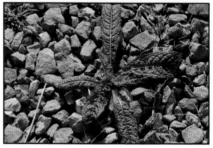

Michael Tierra states "It is used to strengthen the bones and tendons and promote circulation." The doctrine of signatures could point to the bone with the spines contained on the top and bottom of the leaf. Gerard states, "The roots of these plants have a certain cleansing facultie," but then continues to say, "There is small use of Teasel in medicines." I think there is a great need for teasel in herbal medicine!

Teasel is a biennial herb, and therefore, the root needs to be harvested from the first-year plant in the fall. This means the root should be harvested before flowering the second year because the plant dies after it sets seed, and the root is no longer viable for use in herbalism. I wash and chop up the root to use fresh in a tincture. That is the only herbal preparation I have used. You can use drop dose or standard dosing with this herb. I like to start at a lower dose and gradually add more if they are needed.

I have used teasel for both myself and my clients to help with pain and inflammation in the joints and muscles. I started also using this herb as a specific for "aching bones" or bone-deep pain which I believe it has helped those clients. It is beneficial in cases of fibromyalgia syndrome, arthritis, and Lyme disease. I do believe it works as an alterative, cleansing the body of toxins as well, especially through the liver. It has relaxing properties as an antispasmodic and will relieve tension and spasming in the muscles. It has stimulating properties in the reproductive system, the nervous system, the circulatory system, and the digestive system with its pungency and bitter taste.

Exercise

When you have the opportunity, harvest the first-year roots and make a fresh tincture using the folk method with 75 percent alcohol content (pack the jar full of roots and pour 195 proof Everclear ¾ full in the jar and distilled water in the rest). Macerate for 4 weeks, strain, and bottle. Document the taste, actions, and your experiences using drop doses and increasing as needed up to 30 drops, 3 times a day. If you do not have first-year roots, you can purchase a fresh tincture of roots to document the same information.

🌿 Increasing the number of tinctures in your apothecary! Keep going!

Thyme (*Thymus vulgaris*)

Taste: Pungent

Qualities: Warming and drying

Parts used: Herb

Medicinal properties: Anthelmintic, antimicrobial, antioxidant, antiphlogistic, antispasmodic, carminative, diaphoretic, digestive, emmenagogue, expectorant, nervine, stimulant

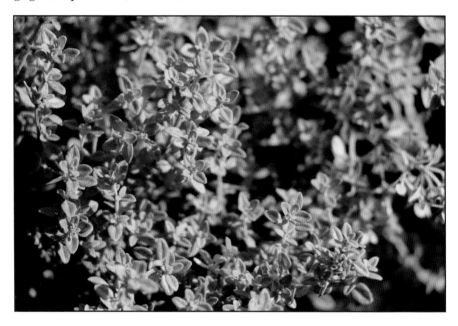

Thyme is a very strong antimicrobial herb as are most of the culinary mints. This antimicrobial strength is demonstrated in Listerine where they use a constituent from thyme to kill germs in the mouth along with others. You will also see thyme being used in many different natural cleaning products. The herb is used for all of the medicinal properties mentioned above.

I grow multiple thyme plants due to their smaller stature for harvesting purposes. I do bring one plant indoors during the winter so that I have fresh leaves for culinary uses. As soon as it grows tall enough, I will begin harvesting from the plant by cutting roughly four to five inches of the stem before flowering. Do not cut too far down so the plant can continue to grow. I like to leave at least five inches of growth on the plant.

Pruning this way encourages more growth for future harvesting. I like to make a fresh tincture with my harvest, and dry the rest for later use in infusions, oils, ointments, steams, fomentations, and baths. Dosages are usually standard with this herb.

Almost everyone has thyme in their kitchen as a spice; however, commercial mints will not be as potent as freshly harvested and dried herb from your own garden. I use thyme in baths and steams as an antispasmodic, antiphlogistic, and expectorant herb. If someone is suffering from nasal or chest congestion, inhaling the steam will reduce inflammation and remove excess mucus from the lungs. Using this pungent and aromatic mint will stimulate the digestive process, remove excess flatulence, increase blood supply to injured connective tissue, stimulate blood flow with menses, and increase perspiration (warm infusion only). As an antispasmodic, it is beneficial with reducing digestive, urinary, or respiratory spasms. Traditionally, thyme was utilized in whooping cough whether taken internally or inhaling the steam. I also use this herb with other anthelmintic and antimicrobial herbs for the digestive system.

Exercise

Try making a steam for nasal congestion next time you are in need. Place the herb in hot water, cover, and let it steep for 20 minutes. Place a towel over your head, take the cover off, and place your nose over the steam at intervals while you inhale the aromatics. What were the results?

🌿 A standard kitchen spice, but potent herbal ally just added to your inventory.

Valerian (*Valeriana officinalis*)

Taste: Bitter and acrid

Qualities: Warming and drying

Parts used: Root

Medicinal properties: Alterative, analgesic, antispasmodic, anxiolytic, carminative, cathartic (large doses), digestive, diuretic, emmenagogue, hepatic, nervine, sedative

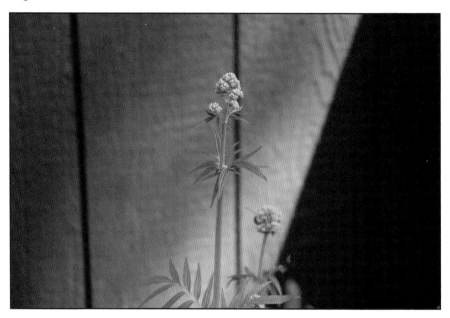

Valerian is a popular sedative herb for those suffering from insomnia. It is one of the first herbs recommended for that condition, but it is not for everyone. There is a small population that valerian causes excitability instead of calming actions in the body. The only way to know if someone is from that small population is for them to ingest the herb. Grown in the garden, you have the ability to use the fresh root in your herbal preparations, but you should be aware of how easily this plant spreads through self-seeding. It is recommended that you cut most of the flowers before they seed to prevent this while leaving a few to replenish your supply. The root is mostly used in herbal preparations, which is what I use, but I have also heard of the leaves being utilized medicinally. Feel free to experiment with the leaves and compare medicinal properties with the root.

I harvest the roots in the fall after the plant dies back for use in a fresh tincture. I dry the herb for later use in other herbal preparations, or to sell in bulk to my clients. Personally, I prefer the tincture over an infusion or decoction because of the smell. The fresh root does not have a rancid smell and the flowers smell absolutely divine, but once the roots dry, valerian has a disagreeable odor that some would compare to dirty socks. I prefer to use drop dosing and move up to standard as needed for a short period of time only. This is not an herb that I want to use in larger doses or for long durations.

Valerian is not the first sedative herb I reach for when I am having trouble sleeping, or when one of my clients is. I like to use valerian when nerve pain accompanies insomnia, or when anxiety is becoming more frequent in an individual. It is a good choice when there is tension, pain, or spasms in the digestive system too along with other nervous or muscular issues. I will also choose valerian as an alterative for kidney and liver stimulation when needed and if it is indicated. I like to use drop dosing during the daytime hours, and standard dosing one hour before bedtime if needed due to its sedative effects. I rarely use this herb as a simple, and I prefer to add it to a formula.

Exercise

If you have the opportunity to grow valerian, you can do this exercise. Harvest the fresh root. Wash and cut it up and smell it at this time. Use it to make a fresh decoction (and a fresh tincture if you can) and save some to dry. As the root is drying, what does it smell like?

Make another decoction with the dried root. Sip this decoction and document the taste and actions on the body. Compare the taste and actions with the fresh decoction and/or tincture. Which do you prefer? What are your preferences? Any differences found?

If you cannot grow valerian, purchase the dried root and a fresh tincture for comparisons.

🌿 *A great herb to add to your apothecary.*

Violet (*Viola* spp.)

Taste: Sweet, slightly bitter, and sour
Qualities: Cooling and moistening
Parts used: Flowers and leaves
Medicinal properties: Alterative, antioxidant, antiphlogistic, antispasmodic, aperient, demulcent, diuretic, emollient, expectorant, lymphatic, nervine, nutritive

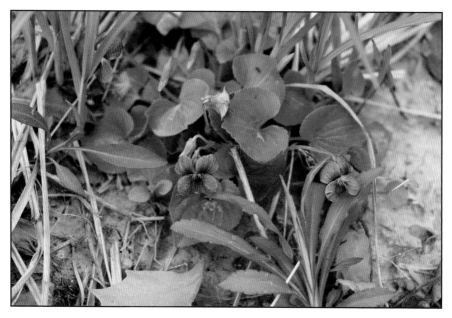

Violets are also called heart's ease for their ability to help release anger while comforting and strengthening the heart. I personally use the blue violet flower essence for releasing anger, and the white violet flower essence for purity of the heart to bring harmony, gratitude, and enjoyment of life to the individual. The flowers and leaves are edible and are used to make baked goods, cocktail beverages, syrup, and jams. The leaves and flowers both provide the aforementioned medicinal properties. This is not a popular herb in commerce, but it is a popular herb amongst herbalists that have experience with it.

I look forward every spring to sit down on the warm ground and pick flowers and leaves for my culinary delights and my medicinal applications. On the first harvest, I make a fresh tincture, fresh syrup, and save some for my salads and baking. The rest of my harvesting throughout the spring is collected for drying for future use as infusions, soothing baths, healing oil, and fomentations. I like to combine the tincture in a formula with other herbs or use it as a simple. I most often combine violet with other herbs when a cooling and moistening nervine is needed to either balance the individual or the herbal formula itself. Standard dosing is mostly used with this herb, but the maximum can be safely utilized when needed.

When I am asked what my favorite herb is, violet makes the list. I like to use an infused oil to reduce inflammation, soothe irritation, and cool the skin. It works great externally on hives, hard lumps, congested lymph system, eczema, acne, mastitis, and is an added benefit in cosmetics for its soothing qualities. I love the tincture as a supportive lymphatic and nervine ally. Its relaxing qualities are used for tension headaches, emotional upheaval, IBS, and other stress related symptoms. It is soothing for inflammatory diseases in the urinary and digestive systems too. I find it a good addition to the diet for its nutritional, antioxidant, and demulcent qualities. Opening the jar of dried flowers and leaves offers an aroma that is reminiscent of joy.

Exercise

There are two parts and two herbal preparations in this exercise. You will first infuse an oil (your choice) with dried violet leaves (or both leaves and flowers) in a double boiler, simmering for about an hour. Strain, cool, bottle, and label. Use this oil externally, add it to cosmetics, or make an ointment by melting beeswax in it. Document your results.

The second exercise includes using the fresh flowers if you are able to harvest some to make a violet simple syrup. Pick the flowers, remove the green calyx and stems, and fill a small jar. Add hot distilled water to this and let it steep overnight. Strain the flowers and add an equal amount of granulated sugar to the liquid. Simmer (do not boil) this until the sugar dissolves. Store this in the refrigerator. Use it in cocktail beverages, icing, or baked goods.

🍃 An herbal base to use alone or add to other remedies just created for your apothecary!

Yarrow (*Achillea millefolium*)

Taste: Bitter and pungent
Qualities: Neutral (can be both warming and cooling) and drying
Parts used: Flowers and leaves
Medicinal properties: Alterative, anodyne, antiphlogistic, antiseptic, anxiolytic, astringent, diaphoretic, diuretic, emmenagogue, hemostatic, hepatic, nervine, stimulant, tonic, vulnerary

Yarrow is considered an ampho-teric herb. This means that it has a normalizing effect on an organ or body system, and it can often have opposite effects on each depending on the need of the body. Yarrow can stop bleeding from a wound or hem-orrhaging after childbirth, but it can also stimulate movement of bleeding if there is current stag-nation. It can be warming or cooling. It can be stimulating to the urinary system as a diuretic

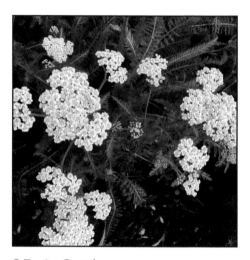

© Denise Cusack

or stop excessive fluid leaking from incontinence. The aerial parts of the plant are used for all of the medicinal properties mentioned above.

I harvest the leaves before the plant begins flowering, and I will col-lect the flowers and leaves as soon as the flowers open. The flowers will produce all season long and you can continue to harvest throughout the growing season if more is needed. I will make a fresh tincture immedi-ately and dry the rest for use in other herbal preparations. I tie a bundle of flowers and leaves together and hang them upside down to dry. The dried parts are used to make warm infusions, oils, ointments, and baths. Either drop dosing or standard dosing is used with this herb as needed.

Yarrow is a must-have plant in the garden, or in your medicine chest. I utilize this herb as a diaphoretic when someone is sick with a cold or flu, as a hemostatic and vulnerary with a wound, as an emmenagogue to stimulate menstruation, as an anodyne for a toothache, as a stimulant to the circulatory system, or when needed to support the body or the individual emotionally when they need courage or strength. I use the flower essence for the individual that needs help breaking out of their shell, or they feel weak, threatened, or subjected. I use the warm infusion, the tincture, and the infused oils mostly in my practice, but I will also use the leaves as a fresh poultice to help stop bleeding or eliminate swelling and pain. I like to include it as a simple, or in my formulas with other herbs. It is included in a popular combination for colds and flus with both peppermint and elderflowers in equal proportions. As a bitter amphoteric, I use it to balance the digestive system.

Exercise

Look up identifying characteristics of yarrow and look for some in your area. Document the type of area you find it growing in. You could also grow some yarrow to complete this exercise. Once you find or have some growing, harvest one leaf and chew it. Notice the taste, actions, and results in your mouth and body after 15 minutes. What did you notice happening?

Research yarrow and write up a list of first aid situations and different herbal applications you would use with this herb for those situations. Is this an herb you wish to have on hand in your home? Do you have enough yarrow growing around you, could you grow some yourself, or do you need a resource to purchase from? Create those herbal preparations!

🌿 An important herb with many applications just added to your apothecary!

Yellow dock (*Rumex crispus*)

Taste: Bitter and sour

Qualities: Cooling with both drying and moistening effects

Parts used: Root

Medicinal properties: Alterative, aperient, astringent, cholagogue, diuretic, hepatic, lymphatic, tonic

Yellow dock is also called curly dock due to the wavy edges of the leaves. It is considered one of the best blood builders and organic sources of iron in nature. The leaves can be used for nutritional purposes with a high content of vitamin A and C, manganese, iron, calcium, phosphorus, magne- 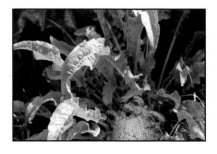 sium, selenium, riboflavin, and thiamine. But due to the oxalate content, it is recommended to boil the leaves, strain and discard the water, then boil in fresh water and strain once more prior to eating.[25] The root is normally the part used medicinally for all of the above medicinal properties.

I like to harvest the roots of yellow dock in the fall once the leaves start to discolor. You will notice the brown flowered stalk of the plant announcing its location. The taproot goes deep into the soil, and it cannot always be dug up whole and will regrow if any root is left. I wash and 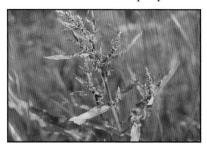 cut the root into smaller pieces for drying later and use some of the fresh root to make a tincture. This is a bitter herb, and it can be combined with other herbs in a formula to help with the taste, or you can make a syrup with the decoction. Just make sure the bitter taste isn't covered up if it is needed for the digestive system. This herb can be used in drop doses, or in standard doses.

In my practice, I utilize this herb in cases of anemia, when there is heavy bleeding in menstruation to supplement the iron lost, with chronic acne or other skin diseases, with kidney or liver stagnation, or when digestive support is needed. Yellow dock helps absorb the nutrients taken in while balancing the digestive secretions. I like to make the syrup to use as a digestive aide and to supplement iron by adding a little less than the 2:1 ratio so more of the bitter taste can still be present, then refrigerate it. I also combine the tincture with other herbal tinctures to create custom formulas for my clients. I particularly like it combined with burdock, ground ivy, or red clover as supporting alteratives.

Exercise

In this exercise, you will make a decoction of the dried roots with a small amount of blackstrap molasses or honey (make a syrup) for use as a nutritive, alterative, and digestive supporting tonic. You will need: 2 ounces dried yellow dock root, a saucepan with lid, 1 quart distilled water, ½ cup blackstrap molasses or raw honey, a bottle with a cap, and a label.

Pulse the root gently in a coffee grinder and place the ground root in the pan with the water. Bring to a boil, then simmer until ½ the volume is left (2 cups). Cover and let simmer for 20 minutes, strain, cool until slightly warm, then add the molasses or honey and stir until it dissolves. Once it is cooled, bottle, label, and place it in the refrigerator for storage.

🌿 Congratulations for adding another herbal remedy to your apothecary!

Chapter Twenty-Two
Choosing the Right Herb

Learning to pick the right herb for the right person takes some practice, and it includes a process of combining the knowledge of the medicinal properties of the herb, the energetics of the herb, the energetics of the individual, and the needs of the individual. This might sound like a lot to remember or think about, but you will get better the more you practice and the more experience and knowledge you have with each herb.

Mary's Advice
Your journals will be a good reference for you in the future when you research information about an herb. You can refer back to your journals for your own personal experiences with them along with how you used each and at what doses. Priceless information for you!

In Chapter Eighteen (page 92), I gave you steps on how to combine medicinal properties and energetics using the knowledge I gave you prior to that chapter. The exercise given in that chapter asked you to choose five people experiencing different symptoms around you. You were to determine the medicinal properties needed for each individual, and then determine the energetics of the five individuals along with the plant energetics needed to balance them. You will need to retrieve that exercise to complete the exercise below.

In Chapter Nineteen (page 97), I explained how to use the herb section of this book. I had asked you to take the time to research each herb individually before you completed each exercise. This could include contraindications and interactions, any scientific studies done on the herb, history and folklore of each herb, its growing conditions and identification, possibly other plants that could be mistaken for the herb, and what other experiences herbalists have documented about each herb. This is important additional information you need in order to solidify your knowledge of each herb and be able to choose the correct herb in any given situation.

The information provided about each herb included some of my own experiences. After research and your own personal experiences with each, you might decide on other uses for the herb, decide on different energetics for each herb, and decide on different herbal preparations to make with each herb. You might have different philosophies regarding how you want to practice herbalism that don't reflect mine, and that is perfectly fine. Ask a number of herbalists which herb they choose for an individual or what preparation they prefer, and you will get a number of different herbs and choices of preparations. Are they wrong? No, they aren't. Every herbalist has their favorite herbs to work with, and how they like to use them. If the herb matches the individual's need and energetics and helps them, that is all that matters. There are so many different herbs than the ones I have written about in this book, and it is my hope you will continue studying and researching new herbs as you grow as an herbalist.

Now that you know the steps, have researched and learned about each of the herbs, and had some experience working with them, let's move on to choosing the right herb. The following exercise at the end of this chapter sets up a thoughtful process for you to follow in choosing the right herb for an individual. You might find that you have more than one herb that will suffice for the situation and the person needing it. Let's take a look at what you can do in this scenario.

All herbs have multiple actions in varying degrees, and it helps to know which herb has a stronger medicinal property, or which organs the herb has an affinity for. Think back to historical uses with each herb and their possible indications (a symptom, type of person, or special situations for the use of a particular herb gathered from personal experience or study) that can further help you decide on the correct herb out of the possible selections. Here are some additional steps that I may take when deciding on the right herb out of multiple choices in my pantry for my clients.

1. Think about the strength of each herb for the medicinal properties needed. Is one stronger than the other in action?

2. Look at which organ the herbs have an affinity for. Compare it to the needs of the individual.
   a. As an example: You need an antispasmodic herb, and each of your choices have the correct energetics needed. If one of the herb's affinity organs is the lungs and the other herb's affinity organ is the digestive system, the choice will be easy to make if your client has coughing spasms.
3. Look at the historical and traditional uses of an herb to help you decide on the best choice.
   a. As an example: Red clover was traditionally used in whooping cough. This might be the right herb for the coughing spasms in your client rather than catnip (*Nepeta cataria*), which is also an antispasmodic but was not necessarily used traditionally in that manner.
4. Look at the indications for each herb that you would find in your research, or you have noticed in your own experiences.
   a. As an example: Passionflower (*Passiflora incarnata*) is indicated for the individual that cannot quiet their mind before sleeping and cannot fall asleep compared to blue vervain (*Verbena hastata*), which is indicated in the individual characterized by Matthew Wood in *The Earthwise Herbal* as "strong above and weak below." Does the individual have trouble shutting down their thoughts, or are they the type that makes a list and has a low libido? This could help in the choice.
5. Will you be using this herb for a longer period of time? If so, which one is a tonic or trophorestorative herb and can be safely used for longer durations?
6. Does one herb interact with any medications the individual is on or contraindicate with any health conditions they might have? Safety first!

These are just some other possible steps that you can think through in order to know you have chosen the best selection for the individual. You might still come up with more than one herb to choose from out of your pantry after following these steps, and in that case, either would be fine to use.

PART SIX

Basic Needs of the Apothecary

Chapter Twenty-Three
Shelf Expectancy

The shelf life of an herb or herbal preparation should be considered when you are purchasing either from a supplier. This is also an important consideration to keep in mind in the apothecary. Our herbal preparations are only as good as the quality of the herbs that we make them with, along with how they are extracted and stored. Shelf expectancy refers to how long an herb or herbal preparation has been stored on a shelf and relies on the age of the herb, how they are prepared, the menstruum used, the containers they are in, and where they are stored.

When I mention the age of the herb, I am not talking about the age of the plant. I am referring to how long ago the plant was harvested. A plant is only fresh until the water content has evaporated, which in turn will make the plant dried. At this point, it is important to know how long that dried herb has been stored because certain herbs lose potency after drying, exposure to the air, and after a certain period of time goes by.

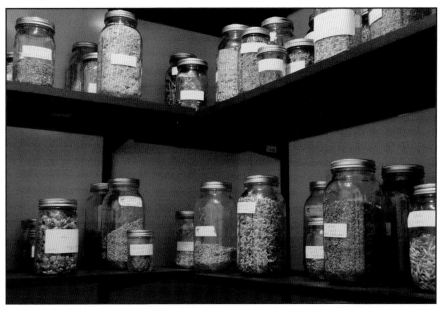

The quality of an herbal preparation can be determined by how soon an herb is processed, and how an herb is prepared will determine the shelf life. Do you plan to use it fresh? If that is the case, the herb should be processed within a day of harvesting (unless it is in water and refrigerated). If you plan to use it dried, the herb should be processed within one year of proper storage. There are times when I will test my herb for potency if they are older than one year. If it is an aromatic herb and it still has a strong fragrance, I will keep using it. If you plan on powdering the herb, they should be used in a preparation immediately, or stored properly no longer than one year. Some herbs lose potency quickly once they are powdered, so it is best to know the herb before grinding them.

Which type of menstruum is used in the herbal preparation determines the shelf life of a product. Here is a list of herbal preparations with their shelf expectancy:

- **Tinctures**: The potency of an alcoholic extract will last a good seven years or more. As far as going bad or spoiling, always smell and listen for a pop when you open the cap of a bottle. For the most part, alcohol kills bacteria; however, if a lower amount of alcohol than recommended is used (or it's prepared improperly), the preparation could spoil. I rarely use a tincture older than five years because I like to make it fresh for my business, but it's not necessary to do this.

> ### Mary's Advice
> A good practice is keeping documentation of the date each herbal preparation was made to determine when it needs to be replaced in the apothecary, or put the date on each bottle label.

- **Infusion/decoction**: All full water extracts should be made daily and not kept on a shelf for longer than that day. If you want to make a bigger batch, you can add alcohol or vegetable glycerin for preservation. Some herbs such as licorice root (*Glycyrrhiza glabra*) are best made for storage as a tincture by making a decoction first and then adding at least 40 percent alcohol. If enough alcohol is used, it will last like a tincture. You can also add 50 percent vegetable glycerin to the infusion/decoction based on the volume of the liquid made for months of storage.

- **Glycerites**: On the other hand, if 100 percent of vegetable glycerin is used to extract a fresh herb, or at least 60 percent glycerin is used to extract a dried herb, you will get about three years of shelf life if it is stored properly. Some herbalists like to make them yearly (I am one of those).
- **Acetum/vinegars**: A vinegar herbal preparation will last for six months if stored properly.
- **Oils/salves**: An oil infusion will last for up to one year when stored properly.
- **Succus**: This preparation doesn't last long by itself. For shelf stability, I will add at least 40 percent alcohol to it.
- **Infused honey**: If dried herbs are used to infuse the honey, shelf life is roughly one year for potency, and they do not need to be refrigerated. However, if fresh herbs or berries are used, the honey could ferment, and the consistency will be thinner. I prefer to use dried herbs to infuse my honey. If fresh herbs are needed, I will make smaller amounts that I can refrigerate for three months at a time.
- **Syrups**: The shelf expectancy of an herbal syrup will depend on the ratio of water and honey used. If you use a 1:2 ratio (one part infusion/decoction to two parts honey), it can be used within the year if it is refrigerated; otherwise, shelf life is three months.
- **Electuaries**: Powdered herbs mixed into honey have a shelf life between six months and a year while refrigerated.

Containers can be as much fun as they are necessary. Not only that, the type of container you choose can make a difference in shelf expectancy of your herbal preparations. There are many different shapes, colors, sizes, and material to choose from; however, the most important aspect of your container should be color when it comes to shelf life. Storage of these containers should be in a cold dark area and each container should be airtight. Clear glass containers will let in light, which can either cause heat or oxidation, resulting in the loss of potency. I store my dried herbs in a dark closet in large mason jars. I choose a brown or blue container for all of my tinctures, bottles, and jars to keep out as much light as possible. Keeping the light from reaching your herbs or herbal preparations is key to reaching full potential of shelf expectancy.

Chapter Twenty-Four
Standard Inventory in the Apothecary

The complete apothecary contains both an inventory of material that will be used to create herbal preparations, and the finished products prepared ahead of time that will be needed in the future for different situations. Throughout this book, there have been exercises to help you start assembling some of these herbal preparations already. I previously spoke about tools of the trade, and I gave you a checklist of tools and other material that will be used to make these products when creating your apothecary. I have also prepared you to learn, research, and experiment with thirty-five different herbs that will make a nice assortment of medicinal properties to include in it. Hopefully, you have taken the time to work with these herbs detailed in Chapter Twenty-One (page 102). If not, please do so before you begin Part Seven of this book (page 197). This chapter details the types of herbal preparations you will need to prepare to be included in this inventory along with other helpful additions that will benefit your home apothecary.

In the apothecary, shelf expectancy is something you want to keep in mind as you are thinking about the different kinds of herbal preparations you want, and how often you want to prepare them. It will be a good idea to have each of the thirty-five herbs in their dried form. I keep mine in an airtight container located in the closet on shelves, and they are alphabetized for easier accessibility. You will use these dried herbs for making infusions, decoctions, baths, steams, fomentations, and syrups for immediate use as needed and for any other extracts that will take time to make. They are also important to have on hand to make any herbal preparations that are in need of replenishing. Eventually, the trick will be to harvest/purchase just enough of the herbs to get you through a typical year of usage. Obviously, this will take experience and time to get better at determining how much is needed.

It will also be a good idea to have each of the thirty-five herbs made into a tincture for three reasons:

1. Shelf expectancy of seven or more years
2. Convenience of dosing
3. Convenient in formulating and creating custom tinctures with multiple herbs for an individual

Mary's Advice

Learning about solubility and phytochemistry is an additional in-depth category of herbalism to learn. You can look up information and training in this subject at any time.

When researching each herb, you will find out whether or not they are water or alcohol soluble. Each herb contains multiple chemical constituents that you will find are best extracted by either water or alcohol. Some herbs containing mucilage will be tinctured with less alcohol, some containing resins will need a higher amount of alcohol, and some water-soluble herbs will be best made into a decoction with added alcohol for preservation. Before you make each tincture, research how to tincture each herb, and you will find the correct way of making them. You can also research a menstruum chart to find out how much alcohol is used to make each herb into a tincture.

I personally like to have tinctures on hand so that I can create a convenient way of dosing and formulating for my clients. Not everyone likes to make or drink an infusion/decoction, and not everyone has the time to make them. However, if you are from an alcohol-free home and you wish to avoid tinctures and alcohol completely, you can make alternatives for medicine. It is always best to have another way to deliver the medicinal properties of an herb for those that cannot have alcohol, or at the very least be able to offer it to them. This could mean the difference in how soon the individual can begin the herb if you don't have enough of the dried herb for their use, or they need a special extract made that doesn't use alcohol. When using alternatives, you will not have the shelf expectancy that alcohol gives, but you will still receive some of the same benefits. You could make glycerites (the dosage is double that of tinctures), acetums (don't extract every constituent), herbal honeys, infusions, decoctions, electuaries, or even apply external applications of herbs to get the same medicine. There can be differences in the amount of herb used, how often they are replenished or made, how much of a dose is administered, and how frequent each dose is administered with each different alternative herbal preparation that is used. I know quite a few herbalists that are alcohol-free and are very adept at their craft.

Remember when I told you not every herbalist is the same? This includes their philosophies and the way they prepare and apply herbs. Not only do herbalists have favorite herbs, they also have favorite ways of using them. So, this is where you can take the time and decide which herbal preparations you would like to prepare and use in your own apothecary. You could also research the philosophies of other herbalists to help you decide which way is right for you and your apothecary.

Whether or not you choose to make a tincture of every one of the thirty-five herbs to have on hand in your apothecary, you must consider the other types of herbal preparations you will need for emergency uses or as first-aid applications. I like to think ahead about the possible scenarios where the medicinal properties are needed right away, and the individual can't wait to prepare it. Some examples would be for wounds, symptoms of cold/flu, ear pain, muscle spasms, injuries, insect bites, allergies, etc. You can make a list and decide if you want to use single herbs, or a formula. You can also decide if you will use the fresh/dry herbs in an herbal preparation to be made as each situation arises, or if you want something already made to grab immediately.

Exercises

1. Harvest or purchase any herbs from Chapter Twenty-One (page 102) that you haven't been able to get yet.
2. Decide where you will be storing your herbs, tools, ingredients, and herbal preparations.
3. Store your dried herbs correctly.
4. If you plan on making all thirty-five tinctures, research each herb and check the menstruum charts for the correct percentage of alcohol to be included in the menstruum.
5. Make a list of symptoms or conditions that you might encounter and decide what herb or herbs you would like to use along with what herbal preparations would be best to use in these situations. Add the herbs and herbal preparations by each on this list.
6. Use this list to decide what you will add to your apothecary from the exercises and herbal formulas available.
7. Prepare all the tinctures you haven't finished yet.

🌿 You now have a convenient form of herbal medicine in your apothecary!

Chapter Twenty-Five
Checklist before Proceeding

You have come a long way since the beginning of this book. You have learned the basics of herbalism, researched thirty-five herbs (plus more) and studied them, experimented with those herbs, and started building your own home apothecary. Before going to Part Seven, take the time to ensure that you have all the supplies, herbs, and herbal preparations ready as you move forward.

- Go back to Chapter Twelve (page 54) and make sure you have everything on that list.
- Stock all of the thirty-five herbs in your apothecary if you haven't already (and others that you have researched).
- Make sure you have been able to do all the exercises in this book.
- Prepare the other herbal preparations throughout this book if you haven't already done so (except the ones containing alcohol if that needs to be avoided).
  - Lavender and rosemary spray oil (page 15)
  - Flower essences (page 16)
  - Calendula bolus (page 59)
  - Garlic oil (page 61)
  - Fire cider (page 215)
- Finish making the thirty-five tinctures if you choose.

At this point, you should have all of your journals finished to act as a reference guide along with this book. Keep writing in your journals, and eventually you will have your own home remedies to hand down with dos and don'ts, dosages, instructions, and ingredients. You will also have journals containing harvesting instructions for the plants around you, journals with the optional flower essences you created, and journals for each herb that you have connected with. These are your stories to tell.

One more idea for another journal would be to use it as a questions and answer book. Write your questions down when you have one, research the answer, and write the answer underneath the question. This will help you as a teacher and as an herbalist.

Exercise

This is as good a time as any to get started on asking questions and looking for the answers. I am sure you have some, and as a student self-studying at home, you are your best teacher.

Purchase or make a separate journal for these questions and answers and fill your mind! Remember that I will have resources for you in Chapter Thirty-One. This will give you places to look for those answers.

PART SEVEN

Herbal Preparations and Remedies

Chapter Twenty-Six
More Herbal Preparations and Formulas for the Apothecary

Previously, I asked you to make a list with the health situations you might come across in the near future and write down the herb(s) you would like to use along with the type of herbal preparation you preferred to make with that herb. You might try your hand at creating your own formulas or recipes, or you can look at the following formulas in this chapter using some of the thirty-five herbs highlighted in this book and decide if you would like to make them instead. The exercises in the previous chapters had you create different herbal preparations that you could use to create some of the following formulas. It is possible to combine separate herbal preparations to create a new formula such as an herbal honey and a tincture (elixir), or a tincture with an infusion.

Mary's Advice
Another subject you can learn about is formulating with herbs if you are interested in creating your own products or formulas. It is a good skill to have in herbalism.

When you combine different types of herbal preparations, there are a few things to keep in mind that could affect the integrity of your final product. They are:

• **Water and oil do not mix**. You cannot mix herbal preparations that contain oil with others that contain water. They just won't mix. An example would be an essential oil added to an infusion, or a decoction mixed with an infused oil.

- **Shelf expectancy could change**. Using dried herbs to infuse in honey has a shelf-life of one year, but if you decide to combine a water-based extract to this, the shelf expectancy could be reduced (such as a syrup).
- **The way you store it could change**. Dried infused herbal honeys can be stored in a cabinet, but if water is added to it, refrigeration might be needed.
- **Consistency could change**. Adding water to honey will thin the consistency.
- **Taste could change**. Combining different herbal preparations will also affect the taste of the final product. Does the combination enhance the flavor of the herbal preparation or change it to disagreeable taste?
- **Is this combination necessary**? Could you get the same medicinal actions using each of the herbal preparations separately? The infusion could be taken separately from the tincture for example. What is the purpose of combining each of them? Decide what is more convenient for the individual.

Another thing to keep in mind are the medicinal properties and energetics included in each herbal preparation. This will be important for you to remember when choosing the right one for both the situations and the individuals that need it. You can review previous chapters as a reference. For example, you should have on hand different expectorant herbal preparations or individual herbs that are balancing for the different constitutions or tissue states of each individual. Coughs and respiratory issues could be either drying or moistening. You will want to choose the right expectorant herb in this situation to balance those energetics.

In my home and business, I have on hand certain formulas with multiple herbs that are already finished and can be used immediately. Because the following situations tend to come up more often and help for them is usually needed right away, I like to make these herbal preparations ahead of time and have them ready to go. A few of the situations could include:

- Muscle spasms or cramping
- Coughs

- Digestive issues
- Sprains and swelling
- Minor wounds
- Burns
- Rashes

Not every situation will need a combination of herbs. Most of the time, I like to work with formulas consisting of multiple herbs for a wider range of actions to benefit some of these situations. However, sometimes using just one herb is all that is necessary. You will see the use of these in the following herbal preparations I have provided for you.

Each of the formulas or individual herbs will be broken down into the categories of herbal preparations for easier reference. I will explain why each of these would be beneficial in your apothecary and give you the instructions on making them. It will be up to you to research the correct dosages to use with each depending on the herbs used, the type of herbal preparation, and the individuals needing them. (Refer to Chapters Thirteen and Fourteen on pages 59 and 65 for more information.) The fun part is to make the formulas I give you, and then create some of your own. Keep a journal and compare what you like and what you don't like about them, which one works better, and how soon each worked for you. This is beneficial information to have for your apothecary.

Ointments/Oils

Multipurpose ointment: This ointment is an all-purpose external application of herbs with antimicrobial, antifungal, nervine, antiphlogistic, and astringent medicinal properties. Great for wound care, external fungal infections, and nerve pain.

Equal parts of these dried herbs are infused into the Saint-John's-wort oil previously made in Chapter Twenty-One (page 102):

- Black walnut; leaves
- Sweet leaf; leaves and flowers
- Calendula; flowers
- Yarrow; leaves and flowers

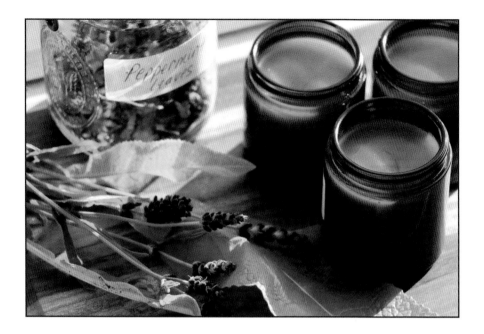

Measure one cup of the Saint-John's-wort oil and place this oil in the top of a double boiler. Place water in the bottom pan. Add roughly four tablespoons of each herb in a separate bowl. Pulse the herbs in a coffee grinder or grind them with a mortar and pestle. Place the herb mixture into the oil and stir. Simmer the oil while it's covered for an hour while stirring occasionally. Strain this into a cheesecloth placed in a strainer overtop of a bowl or glass liquid measuring cup. Once it's cooled, gather the cheesecloth and squeeze out the excess oil into the bowl. Clean and dry the double boiler. Pour the strained oil back into the top of the double boiler, add ¾ ounce beeswax, and simmer until the wax is melted. Pour this liquid into 2 (4-ounce) jars and label them. You can adjust the recipe for additional jars.

🌿 Great job! You just made an ointment that will be used for many different kinds of situations. Refer back to each herb in Chapter Twenty-One (page 102) if you want to review other possible uses.

Tissue ointment: This will be your external go-to healing ointment for connective tissue. This can include repairing and soothing the skin, speeding up the process of healing the connective tissue, reducing swelling and pain of the injured tissue, and soothing insect bites. It has antimicrobial, astringent, cell proliferant, emollient, and antiphlogistic herbs.

Equal parts of these dried herbs are infused in the chickweed oil that was prepared in Chapter Twenty-One (page 102):

- Comfrey; root
- Self-heal; aerial part
- Plantain; leaves

Measure 1 cup chickweed oil and place this oil in the top of a double boiler. Place water in the bottom pan. Add roughly 5 tablespoons of each herb in a separate bowl. Pulse the herbs in a coffee grinder or grind them with a mortar and pestle. Place this herb mixture into the oil and stir. Simmer the oil while covered for an hour while stirring occasionally. Strain this into a cheesecloth that is placed in a strainer overtop of a bowl or glass liquid measuring cup. Once cooled off, gather the cheesecloth and squeeze out the excess oil into the bowl. Clean and dry the double boiler. Pour the strained oil back into the top of the double boiler, add ¾ ounce beeswax, and simmer until the wax is melted. Pour this liquid into 2 (4-ounce) jars and label them. You can adjust the recipe for additional jars.

🌿 You have another multiple herbal remedy handy for immediate use! Review each herb in Chapter Twenty-One (page 102) as well. (Keep in mind that comfrey should not be used on wounds if a possible infection is there. It closes the wound too quickly.)

Muscle rub ointment: I believe everybody needs a first aid muscle rub in their apothecary. This herbal preparation can be made as an oil, or you can add beeswax for an easier application. Any kind of muscle spasm can benefit from the external application of this particular formula. It is a wonderful addition to aid in massage for those strained and tense muscles. I use it with leg cramps, menstrual cramping, tense shoulders, back and neck pain, and other pain caused by inflammation such as arthritis. Cayenne can be an additional herb for you to study since it is not one of the thirty-five herbs in this book.

You will start off with 3 cups olive oil and add the mixture of dried herbs. Part = ¼ cup

- 2 parts mullein; leaves
- 2 parts rosemary; leaves
- 2 parts lavender; leaves, flowers, or both
- 2 parts peppermint; leaves
- 1 part cayenne (*Capsicum spp.*); peppers or powder
- 1 ounce menthol crystals (optional and added after the herbs are infused)

Place the olive oil in the top part of the double boiler and add water to the bottom pan. Mix the herbs and grind them before adding this mixture to the oil. Simmer the oil while it's covered for an hour while stirring occasionally. Strain this into a cheesecloth that is placed in a strainer on top of a bowl or glass liquid measuring cup. Once cooled off, gather the cheesecloth and squeeze out the excess oil into the bowl. Clean and dry the double boiler. Pour the strained oil back into the top of the double boiler, add 2¼ ounces beeswax (this is where you can also add the menthol crystals if you choose), cover, and simmer until melted. Pour this liquid into 6 (4-ounce) jars and label them. You can double the recipe to get 8 jars out of this formula. You could also add drops of lavender, rosemary, or peppermint essential oils to this blend.

🌿 Another ointment added to your apothecary!

Lymphatic oil: There are times that a good lymph oil is needed to move congestion, help with lymph massage, or reduce the swelling of glands. I like lymph oil to be prepared for emergencies such as ear congestion or pain, mastitis, swollen testes, or swollen lymph nodes from an infection.

Start with one cup of the violet oil that was made in Chapter Twenty-One and add each dried herb: Part = ¼ cup

- 2 parts mullein; leaves
- 1 part self-heal; aerial parts

Place the violet oil in the top part of the double boiler and water in the bottom pan. Mix the herbs and then grind them. Add this herb mixture to the oil. Simmer the oil while covered for an hour while stirring occasionally. Strain this into a cheesecloth that is placed in a strainer and laid over a bowl or glass liquid measuring cup. Once cooled off, gather the cheesecloth and squeeze out the excess oil into the bowl. Once this oil is completely cooled, pour it into 1 (8-ounce) bottle and label it.

🌿 You have added lymphatic oil to your apothecary! Congratulations!

Glycerites

Nonalcoholic digestive aid: This is a simple that I use in my own house that adults and children alike will use. It is good to have on hand when you don't have time to make an infusion, you don't want a tincture, are traveling, or are eating out. I personally like to use a variety of peppermint called chocolate mint. I think it has a more gentle and pleasant taste for everyone. It's not as pungent of a flavor. Use this when there is any kind of digestive upset including nausea, intestinal cramping, or gas.

Remember to use 100 percent vegetable glycerin if you are using fresh herbs, and 60 percent vegetable glycerin with 40 percent water for dried herbs when extracting. Gather these ingredients to make this glycerite:

- Fresh or dried peppermint (or chocolate mint); leaves
- Organic vegetable glycerin
- Distilled water (if using dried herbs)
- Small mason jar

If you are using the fresh leaves, pack the mason jar with the herb. Pour the vegetable glycerin into the mason jar to the rim. Use a utensil handle to push out any air pockets and make sure the vegetable glycerin has reached the bottom while covering all of the herb. You can add more if needed. At this point, you can cap the jar and label it. Place it on your counter and shake this daily for 4 weeks. Also, some people like to use gentle heat to extract the herbs quicker and help with the straining process, which is your choice. After maceration, strain the glycerite and bottle it. Be sure to label the bottle.

If you are using the dried leaves, there are a couple different processes. First, only fill the jar halfway with the dried herb and set this aside. The second difference is that you will combine the vegetable glycerin (60 percent) and water (40 percent) before pouring it into the jar. Combine the vegetable glycerin and water and mix until the vegetable glycerin is clear. Pour this menstruum into the jar and fill it to the top. Cap, shake, and label the jar. Again, gentle heat can be used if you choose. Place it on your counter and shake this daily for 4 weeks. Strain the glycerite and bottle it for storage. Be sure to label this as well.

🍃 You have now created a nonalcoholic digestive aide for your apothecary!

Sleep aid: Not everyone wants to drink an infusion or decoction, and not everyone wants an alcoholic extract to help them relax and sleep. This formula is good to have on hand when traveling, to help calm a child, or when you don't want to make an infusion right away. You can also substitute another herbal infusion or decoction for the distilled water to be combined with the vegetable glycerin for additional formulas or medicinal properties.

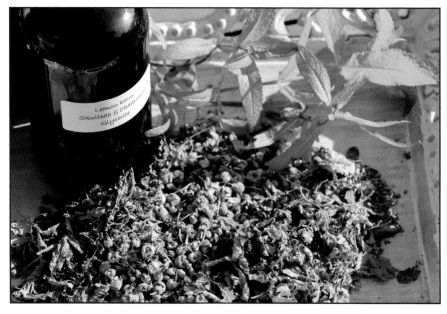

For this herbal preparation, you will combine equal parts of each dried herb. Mix these herbs and add them to a mason jar. For a quart jar: Measurement of equal parts = ¼ cup

- Lemon balm; leaves
- Skullcap; aerial parts
- Chamomile; flowers

Follow the steps for a dried herb glycerite from the nonalcoholic digestive aid instructions prior to this.

🌿 You have completed a sleep aid glycerite for your apothecary that can be used as a base in more formulas in the future.

Throat spray: I can't tell you how many times my family has needed a throat spray to soothe a sore throat. I can send it with each family member, and they can carry it with them as needed. This makes a great gift for others too!

Measure, mix, and grind these herbs to make this herbal preparation. A Part = ⅛ cup for a quart jar.

- 2 parts echinacea; roots
- 2 parts marshmallow; root
- 2 parts plantain; leaves
- 1 part rosemary; leaves

Follow the steps for a dried herb glycerite from the nonalcoholic digestive aid instructions prior to this. You can place the finished glycerite into 1 (4-ounce) bottle with an atomizer to dispense it into the throat. Spray this as needed to soothe the irritated tissue.

🌿 You have completed a throat spray for your apothecary! You will be thankful this is ready to go when you need it.

Herbal Honey

Burn paste: We all hope that this isn't needed but having it on hand to grab quickly makes all the difference in the world. This paste can be directly applied to a burn and covered. Do not rinse this off of a burn.

Continue to add more daily until healed. You can also use this to add to infusions, decoctions, or other beverages. You can also add additional medicine to a tincture and create an elixir.

Gather these ingredients:

- Mason jar
- Dried sweet leaf; leaves and flowers
- Raw unpasteurized local honey

Fill the mason jar halfway with the leaves and flowers. Pour the honey over the herbs slowly until it reaches the bottom of the jar and continue filling to the top. Cap and label the jar, and place this in a sunny window for a month. Strain this at the end of the month (can place in warm water to help with the straining if needed), pour into a jar, cap it, label the jar, and store it for future use.

🌿 You are now prepared for this emergency! Add this to your apothecary!

Herbal Blend for Infusions

Respiratory support: This loose herbal blend is useful for dry coughs. Preparing this blend ahead of time offers demulcent, diaphoretic, expectorant, and antimicrobial properties. It can also be mixed ahead of time and conveniently handed out to family and friends.

Combine equal amounts of each of these dried herbs:

- Violet; leaves only or leaves and flowers
- Marshmallow; leaves, flowers, or both
- Elderflowers

Place these mixed herbs in an airtight container for later use or make loose tea bags and prepare a warm infusion when needed.

🌿 Congratulations on completing these herbal preparations for your apothecary that can be used in first aid situations!

Now that you have all of the thirty-five herbs to work with along with each of these prepared herbal preparations, you have built your apothecary and are ready to add to it! You have a multitude of medicinal properties to utilize for many different types of situations. You have the training and knowledge to use these herbs, and the experience using them will soon follow. All you have to do at this point is add other herbs and herbal preparations as you learn more. Look at the next chapter for some of my favorite remedies that you can prepare too. Keep writing in those journals!

From here, you can research and learn about new herbs to add to your shelves, and experiment with other herbal creations. There are other tools and ingredients that you might find you want to add to your apothecary as well. Continue learning! The last part of this book will include the next steps in learning more about herbalism with other resources to help you on that journey.

Chapter Twenty-Seven
Helpful Remedies

I wanted to include a section in this book that offers some of my favorite remedies. The following formulas will include some new herbs that you haven't learned about yet, harvested, or purchased. This is a great opportunity to take the time to learn what you can about each before obtaining the herb to use in these remedies, which includes any contraindications or interactions they might have. Remember that these might not be good for everyone.

> ### Mary's Advice
> Take a look through these herbal remedies and make a list of the new herbs to study. Which ones grow around you? Will you be growing, wild harvesting, or purchasing them?

Each one of these remedies contains a formula of herbs that can be prepared in different herbal preparations. Throughout this book, I have explained how to create each, and you can review these processes if necessary. I will note which type of herbal preparation I think works the best with each formula. I will also list the main medicinal properties I wanted out of the formula and the possible uses each one can provide. You might find other herbal preparations to make with each formula or find extra uses for each remedy provided that I haven't mentioned. I do have multiple uses for each in my practice. This is why knowing the herbs thoroughly is important. Research the dosing requirements of each herb based on the type of herbal preparation you are creating. You will gain a wealth of knowledge this way and valuable experience using these herbs. Your journals will be a good reference as you gain this experience as well. Practice makes perfect in herbalism.

The Remedies

Respiratory congestion: My go-to internal remedy when mucus is congested in the lungs (stuck phlegm). This is considered to be a damp tissue state or stagnation. This can include sinus drainage into the lungs, allergies, long-standing wet coughs that turn into infections, or coughs that just keep hanging on with some expectoration.

- 2 parts hyssop (*Hyssopus officinalis*); aerial
- 2 parts red raspberry; leaves
- ½ part ginger (*Zingiber officinale*); root

This formula offers the antioxidants and antimicrobial properties needed to help support the immune system during infections or with other invading microorganisms. It also offers antiphlogistic, astringent, and expectorant properties that will be beneficial in reducing inflammatory conditions in the lungs while drawing forth the excess phlegm and expelling it. All of these herbs are drying to balance the excess moisture in the lungs. Hyssop and ginger are considered warming to help stimulate fluid movement and elimination while red raspberry offers antioxidants and cooling energetics to balance this formula.

I think this makes a tasty infusion, but it could also be prepared as a tincture or a glycerite. Combine the formula first before beginning your preferred preparation or save the loose herb mixture for later use. If you already have individual tinctures prepared from each herb, you can combine them together into one bottle. Take the total ounces of the bottle and divide by how many parts there are to the formula. To fill 1 (1-ounce) dropper bottle in this case, you would divide 1 by 4½, which equals .22. Multiply the parts by .22 to get how many ounces to add each tincture to the bottle. You would add .44 ounces each of both hyssop and red raspberry while adding .11 ounces of ginger to 1 (1-ounce) bottle.

Analgesic combination: I love this formula when you want to avoid over-the-counter pain medications. It is just enough to help address some of the causes of pain and reduce the discomfort an individual feels.

- 3 parts mullein; leaves

- 3 parts willow (*Salix* spp.); bark
- 1 part nettle; leaves
- 1 part skullcap; aerial
- 1 part rosemary; leaves

There are many causes of pain, but this formula will address inflammation, muscular tension or spasms, and the nervous system. It offers analgesic, antiphlogistic, relaxing nervine, and antispasmodic medicinal properties that will focus on those causes. Most of the herbs in this formula are cooling except for rosemary. I utilize rosemary as a warming and pungent herb to drive the medicine where it needs to go while offering some of its other medicinal properties. There are also moistening and drying herbs included with this formula.

This combination works well in an infusion although I would decoct the willow bark first and then add the other herbs, cover, and steep. My favorite herbal preparations for this blend would be a tincture or glycerite. You could also use the dried herbs in an oil or ointment for external use. If you have the individual tinctures already prepared, you can easily combine them together into one bottle by measuring out the parts accordingly based on the size of the bottle.

Nourishing blend: This is better than taking any multivitamin! All of these herbs contain a large mixture of micronutrients and macronutrients to nourish the body.

- 2 parts nettle; leaves
- 2 parts oatstraw
- 2 parts red clover; flowers
- 1 part orange peel

These nutrient herbs are beneficial to the entire body and offer antioxidants to support the immune system. Not only does this formula offer nutrition and antioxidants, but it also helps in reducing inflammation, balances the endocrine system, and helps with elimination. This is a very neutral and balancing formula for all energetic qualities.

It would be best to make this formula into an infusion or acetum because both will extract vitamins and minerals more efficiently. You can use either fresh or dried for these, but I usually use dried so I can prepare these throughout the year no matter what the season is.

Clarity of the mind: A well-balanced formula to stimulate and enhance brain function while helping the individual to relax and focus in life. Equal parts of each herb are combined.

- Gotu kola (*Centella asiatica*); leaves
- Sage (*Salvia officinalis*); leaves
- Linden; flowers and bracts
- Schisandra (*Schisandra chinensis*); berries

This formula combines adaptogens and nervines to help with brain fog, memory, stress, and focus. It consists of warming, cooling, drying, and moistening energetics in a balanced formula for all individuals.

I believe the two best herbal preparations to use with this formula would be the tincture or glycerite due to the convenience and how less herbs are used over time. However, an infusion would be appropriate too if you want to take the extra time to prepare it daily. Again, you can either combine all of the herbs together to prepare a tincture, or you can combine the individual tinctures of each herb in one bottle.

Immune support: Instead of always focusing on increasing or modulating the immune system, we should concentrate on preventative care and giving the immune system what it needs to be healthy. Nutrition, sleep, hydration, and exercise all help to keep this body system in good shape. A little extra help in moving and keeping the other body systems in good working order can be beneficial to the immune system as well since they are all interconnected. These include the circulatory, digestive, integumentary, lymphatic, nervous, and respiratory systems.

- 2 parts burdock; root
- 2 parts plantain; leaves

- 1 part rosemary; leaves
- 1 part hawthorn; flowers, leaves, or berries

These herbs contribute nervine, alterative, expectorant, digestive, demulcent, diaphoretic, and stimulant medicinal properties. They aid in the movement of the lymphatic and circulatory system while also stimulating and supporting digestion and acting as a cardiac tonic. Excess heat is released into the periphery of the body through the skin, and tense nerves are relaxed. This formula also contributes to the healing of the mucosal lining in the digestive tract and respiratory system.

I like to make a warm infusion to bring out the diaphoretic property, but the burdock root should first be prepared in a decoction (hawthorn berries, as well, if used). When it is time to steep, I add the rest of the formula to that decoction. This can also be prepared as a tincture or glycerite.

Allergy support: There are different times during the year that certain individuals could use this extra support. This formula helps with common symptoms and slows the release of histamine. If an individual is looking to address the cause of these allergies, then diet and healing of the digestive tract will need to be focused on. Seeking a qualified professional would be beneficial to them. I like to use this formula while addressing the cause.

- 3 parts nettle; leaves
- 3 parts chickweed; aerial
- 2 parts burdock; roots
- 2 parts goldenrod; leaves and flowers
- 1 part plantain; leaves
- 1 part ginger; root

All of these herbs work together to provide alterative, depurant, antiphlogistic, demulcent, hepatic, diuretic, and antiseptic medicinal properties. The alterative and depurant herbs help to facilitate the removal of excess mucus and stimulate the elimination process while the antiphlogistic properties help to reduce the histamine production and reduce the inflammatory process. If mucus remains in these passages for long periods of time, the formation of bacteria and infection could happen. This formula also offers a balance in energetics.

I prefer the infusion of this formula, but I will also make a tincture to take for convenience. A glycerite would also provide the needed medicinal properties from this formula.

Bug repellent spray and oil: This formula isn't necessarily utilized as a medicinal herbal preparation (although it does provide its own medicinal benefits). It does, however, come in handy for the herbal apothecary and for outdoor activities. To make a bug deterring fragrant oil instead, infuse any type of oil with the dried feverfew flowers and add the essential oils once the herb is strained. This oil can be directly rubbed into the exposed skin. It can also be worn as perfume. Here are the ingredients for the spray:

- Feverfew (*Tanacetum parthenium*); flowers
- Vegetable glycerin
- Distilled water
- Witch hazel extract (I get mine from Mountain Rose Herbs)
- Essential oils: rosemary, lemongrass, clove, cinnamon, and lavender

The spray is water-based, but the vegetable glycerin acts as an emulsifier to dilute or blend the water and oils. First prepare one cup of a strong infusion made with feverfew and distilled water. I like to steep these for 40 to 50 minutes. From here, you will separately add ten drops each of the essential oils to one ounce of vegetable glycerin and mix well. This will be very fragrant (which is the point), but it smells divine. Add two ounces of the infusion along with an ounce of witch hazel extract to this mixture and mix again until it is thoroughly blended. Pour this mixture into 1 (4-ounce) glass bottle with an atomizer.

My fire cider blend: There are so many different formulas of fire cider available for the general public with a simple search online. If you haven't already from the Chapter Sixteen exercise (page 87), be sure to research the medicinal benefits of fire cider, the amounts to take, and the contraindications and interactions of the ingredients. I have perfected this particular blend for both myself and my family according to our own tastes, preferences, and medicinal needs. You can make this and experiment along with other recipes to find your favorite. Use organic produce and herbs if you can for this recipe. You will need (approximate measurements):

- Mason jar with lid (one quart)
- Organic apple cider vinegar
- 2 garlic bulbs (fresh cloves either peeled and cut or smashed with removed peel)
- 1 small to medium onion (sliced)
- 1 large ginger root (fresh root, sliced, or dried, cut)
- 3–4 cayenne peppers (fresh or dried, cut); I use Joe's Long Cayenne Peppers
- ½ cup elderberries (dried)
- ¼ cup sweet leaf (dried)
- ½ lemon (sliced)
- Honey for taste

Layer each of these herbs in the jar starting with the garlic cloves, and after each additional herb, press them down in order to fit all of it into the jar. Adjust the amounts of each herb if needed. Once the jar is packed, add the apple cider vinegar and fill it to the top of the jar. Cover the top of the jar with plastic wrap or parchment paper, and then place the lid tightly. Make sure that the jar is labeled with the date and name of the herbal preparation and shake this daily for one month. I leave mine on the kitchen counter out of direct sunlight for this process. At the end of the month, strain the herbs from the liquid and then measure the amount of liquid left. I measure and add honey in half the amount of liquid and mix it very well. You can add the amount you wish according to your own personal tastes.

"Shattered Nerves": This particular blend of herbs benefits the entire nervous system. It is for those suffering from chronic stress, or those that need healing of nerve damage. It feeds the nervous system while it also relaxes tension and stress. This is a blend for when an individual is at their breaking point both physically and emotionally. Part = ¼ cup in the following formula using four cups of distilled water to start:

- 3 parts oats; milky tops
- 2 parts linden; flowers and bracts
- 1 part holy basil (*Ocimum sanctum*); leaves
- ¼ part prickly ash (*Zanthoxylum americanum*); bark (½ part instead if you need more of the analgesic property)

This formula provides stimulant, nervine, trophorestorative, analgesic, antispasmodic, and adaptogen medicinal properties. This combination benefits not only the nerves, but also the heart in a combination of circulatory and muscular health. This is another balanced formula energetically combining warm, cool, moist, and dry herbs.

I will take this in either a decoction, tincture, or glycerite. A vinegar won't extract all of the constituents that are needed. Begin by making a decoction of the oats and prickly ash, and add in the remaining herbs during the steeping process (cover). If you have the individual tinctures already prepared, you can combine them together in one bottle measured accordingly based on the parts. You can also combine this formula into one jar to make a tincture or glycerite.

Cardiovascular support: I like this blend to support the heart muscles, lower cholesterol, stimulate circulation, and help with relaxation. It not only supports the cardiovascular system, but it will also move the lymphatic system and enhance brain function. Combine these herbs together:

- 2 parts hawthorn; leaves, flowers, berries, or a combination
- 2 parts violet; leaves and flowers, or just leaves
- 1 part rosemary; leaves

This formula offers antispasmodic, cardiovascular tonic, stimulant, nervine, hypotensive, and antiphlogistic properties. It is a soothing and great-tasting blend that offers many benefits. Energetically, it is cooling for the most part with a pungent herb used as a catalyst to deliver the medicine where it needs to go. These are usually warming and stimulating herbs that are added to the formula in a small percentage to help deliver and guide the medicine.

I love the taste of this as an infusion, syrup, tincture, or glycerite. My favorite of all is the infusion using both the hawthorn leaves and flowers. I will use the hawthorn leaves, flowers, or berries when making a tincture or glycerite depending on either the availability for harvesting or the availability on my shelves.

Be joyful blend: This formula feeds the body and lifts the heart, so the individual is able to feel joy. An individual's nutrition is addressed while the effects of tension and stress are relieved. Nutrition, toning, strengthening, balancing, and calming are the foundations of this blend with some additional emotional support. The formula consists of:

- 2 parts nettle; leaves
- 2 parts skullcap; aerial parts
- 1 part calendula; flowers
- 1 part rose; petals
- 1 part linden; flowers and bracts

This blend offers relaxing nervine, nutritive, digestive, antiphlogistic, antidepressant, anxiolytic, and antispasmodic properties. Taken internally throughout the day, this formula will help to calm the spirit, the mind, and the body. It is also an uplifting blend to see the brighter side of things. Energetically, this combination consists of mostly cooling and drying herbs with neutral and moistening herbs to help balance each other.

The best way to prepare this formula is with a water extract if you want to get the nutritional benefits. You can prepare a larger batch daily if needed and divide the doses throughout the day. You could also make this into an iced tea after making the warm infusion for those that do not like hot beverages. You can also make this into a tincture if you are getting your nutrition elsewhere and just need the other medicinal properties.

Menstrual support: This herbal remedy focuses on those that suffer from painful menstruation, unbalanced and irregular cycles, and those that need extra emotional support through this particular time. This herbal remedy combines equal parts:

- Yarrow; flowers or leaves and flowers
- Motherwort; aerial
- Red raspberry; leaves
- Holy basil; leaves

This blend will offer emmenagogue, antispasmodic, circulatory, astringent, tonic, anxiolytic, antidepressant, and nervine medicinal properties to support menstruation and any symptoms that can arise during that time. This formula contains mostly cooling and drying herbs with holy basil being considered both warming and neutral.

My favorite herbal preparations with this formula are either a tincture or a glycerite. A syrup could be made from the infusion, or an elixir from the tincture to help improve the taste. It is best to start taking this formula a few days before menstruation for any symptoms, and smaller doses every day until the cycle is regulated. Be sure to know if pregnancy is a possibility first before using it since it contains herbs that are not recommended during that time.

Lactation support: Every mother needs a little support now and then as they are nursing their child. This formula contributes both nutrition and relaxation while also stimulating the milk supply. This formula includes:

- 3 parts blessed thistle (*Centaurea benedicta*); aerial parts
- 3 parts nettle; leaves
- 2 parts red raspberry; leaves
- 2 parts oatstraw
- 2 parts alfalfa (Medicago sativa); leaves
- 1 part hops (*Humulus lupulus*); strobiles

These herbs contribute galactagogue, nervine, and nutritive medicinal properties to this formula. Nutrient deficiencies and stress can make nursing difficult, but this formula helps in both of those areas. This remedy offers mostly cool along with a good balance between dry and moistening energetics, but for those that need a little more warmth, ½ part cinnamon (*Cinnamomum verum*) bark can be added to this blend.

I prefer to use this herbal remedy as an infusion due to its nutritive properties. Water is used to extract vitamins and minerals. Vinegar will extract them too, but it will not extract the other medicinal properties in this formula. If a tincture is preferred, make sure there is 50 percent water content in there. A glycerite can also be made with dried ingredients using 40 percent water.

Digestive support: This remedy has similar uses as the nonalcoholic digestive aid that was in the last chapter, but it also includes additional gentle eliminative balance and digestive support. I use this for children, adults, or the elderly whenever the need arises. It does help with nausea, intestinal and stomach cramping, motion sickness, constipation, diarrhea, and flatulence. This blend combines these herbs:

- 2 parts spearmint (*Mentha spicata*); leaves
- 2 parts raspberry; leaves
- 1 part catnip; leaves
- 1 part chicory (*Cichorium intybus*); root
- 1 part elecampane (*Inula helenium*); root

I find this to be a valuable addition to my apothecary, and you could also prepare this to have in your apothecary for when the need arises. This blend offers digestive, aperient, astringent, and antispasmodic medicinal properties to benefit these situations. These herbs provide mostly cool and dry energetics, but elecampane is added for a pungent and slightly warming effect to move digestion along. Elecampane also brings in prebiotics (inulin) to support a healthy gut flora. For the most part, I enjoy this blend in a tincture or glycerite since they can be easily carried with you to have on hand when needed. The glycerite is my favorite for children or for those that cannot have alcohol.

Liver and kidney support: Sometimes the body can benefit from a formula that helps improve movement of the liver and kidneys. Often, this is a combination of liver, kidney, and gallbladder function improvement. This helps in the removal of waste, balance of hormones, regulation of fluid levels and pH levels in the body, and storage of vitamins and minerals to just name a few. It is much more than detoxification, and I like to refer to this as support for the function of these organs instead. Combine these herbs:

- 2 parts dandelion; root
- 1 part burdock; root
- 1 part marshmallow; root
- 1 part ground ivy; aerial parts
- ¼ part ginger; root

This blend contributes hepatic, diuretic, digestive, tonic, antiphlogistic, cholagogue, demulcent, and stimulant properties to help support these organs. It helps to stimulate movement, increase output of secretions, tone, and strengthen the entire digestive tract. It is beneficial for removing heavy metals, reducing inflammation, repairing the digestive tract, and introducing prebiotics to the gut. There is a good balance of energetics contained in this formula.

I have prepared this remedy in a decoction (ground ivy is added in the steeping process), tincture, and glycerite. I personally prefer to avoid covering some of the bitter taste with sweeteners because the bitter taste has a big effect on the liver and the digestive system. I only use the glycerite if absolutely necessary for a client.

Antimicrobial eyewash: I use this remedy when there is an infection in the eye for both humans and animals. The berberine in this formula is a potent antimicrobial used for conjunctivitis. Originally, I would use goldenseal (*Hydrastis canadensis*) for this purpose because that is the herb I was taught; however, that is an at-risk plant and I prefer to use an alternative herb for this purpose. This remedy includes equal parts:

- Barberry (*Berberis vulgaris, B. thunbergia*); root or twigs
- Raspberry; leaves

This blend not only offers antimicrobial actions, but it also contributes astringent and refrigerant properties. This means in addition to being antimicrobial, it will also offer a drying and cooling sensation to the eyes that is quite refreshing.

To use as an eyewash, you first need to sterilize the eye wash cup (or shot glass). One for each eye is recommended. After making the decoction of barberry root, add the raspberry leaves in the steeping process, and be sure to strain it twice. Pour the liquid remaining into each eye wash cup and let it cool. Once the decoction cools, the eye can be washed by placing the cup to the eye and tilting the head back. Use an old towel or paper towel to catch any drips and be sure to move the eye around for the best coverage. For young children or animals, dip a cotton ball into the decoction, tip the head back, and squeeze the liquid into the corner of the eye. It might be necessary to open the eyelid briefly if they are closing them.

Mouthwash and gargle: This remedy is introduced for daily use to tone and strengthen the gums, reduce bacteria, eliminate bleeding, and reduce inflammation in the mouth and throat. It will need to be made every morning and used throughout the rest of the day. You can prolong the shelf life by adding ⅛ the volume of vegetable glycerin and store it in the refrigerator for three days. Make a water infusion with equal parts of these herbs:

- 2 parts garden sage (*Salvia officinalis*); leaves
- 1 part yarrow; leaves and flowers
- ½ part orange peels

This combination is analgesic, styptic, antiphlogistic, astringent, and antimicrobial. You could use a tincture in water, but it could cause some stinging if there are open wounds in the mouth. Swish the infusion around in the mouth after brushing the teeth and flossing.

Soothing skin wash: This remedy is used externally to promote healing by introducing new skin growth, reducing inflammation, and helping to soothe irritated skin. This can be a beneficial remedy for rashes, eczema, psoriasis, or even chronic dry skin. Combine equal parts of these herbs:

- Chickweed; aerial parts
- Self-heal; aerial parts
- Red clover; flower

These herbs have emollient, antiphlogistic, cell proliferant, and antimicrobial properties that offer a multitude of benefits for the skin when used externally. This remedy can be used to help with symptoms that stem from many different causes, most of which start with diet and the digestive system. So, while relieving the symptoms gets immediate relief, it would be best to combine this remedy with a protocol that addresses the cause. An appointment with a qualified holistic practitioner would help with that. This blend has a cooling and moistening energetics for those hot and inflamed skin conditions.

There are multiple ways to prepare this remedy. An infusion could be made and poured into a warm bath, used as a wash, or used with a fomentation for a specific area. I would also use this as an ointment to carry with me when needed.

All-purpose bath: This blend is aromatic, relaxing, and has a multitude of medicinal properties that it can provide. You can also mix other aromatic herbs into this blend to create a whole new aromatherapy experience. This remedy includes equal parts:

- Chamomile; flowers
- Yarrow; aerial parts
- Calendula; flowers

This blend includes antimicrobial, emollient, antiphlogistic, astringent, antispasmodic, cell proliferant, nervine, and vulnerary medicinal properties. There are many different uses for this blend such as respiratory congestion, tension, fungal infections, nerve pain, poor circulation, arthritis, spasms, achy muscles, colds/flu, or even hemorrhoids. This remedy also lifts the spirit and energizes the body when needed. You can add Epsom salts to this blend or to the bath itself for additional benefits.

Chapter Twenty-Eight
Using the Apothecary

Now that you have created your apothecary, you will need to keep it productive and sanitized throughout the year. There will be times that herbs need to be restocked, supplies need to be replenished, and a thorough cleansing needs to take place. Just as you would keep your kitchen stocked and cleaned, you would need to do the same for the apothecary. There are steps to keep you on track and an assortment of different ways to accomplish this. I will offer some advice and possible ways to manage these tasks below.

Keep the apothecary organized, cleaned, and sanitized. This is the most important step that I believe you can take for the apothecary.

> ### Mary's Advice
> Alphabetize all of the bulk herbs and each of the completed herbal preparations when you are storing them. This makes it easier to find each when they are needed.

- **Organize**: Have a place for everything, and everything put in its place. It is best to know exactly where you put the supplies and herbs so they can be found immediately. There is nothing worse than not being able to find a certain herbal preparation, or not being able to find the cheesecloth because it wasn't put back where it should be. By organizing, you will have an easier time of checking on your supply needs, as well as having what you need in reach when necessary.
- **Cleaning**: Personally, I cannot be creative in a cluttered space. I need to have a clean area to work in and the space to do it. Each person is different in how they work best, but it is imperative that you start with clean supplies and a clean space for sanitary purposes. Clean up after every herbal preparation is produced by washing the supplies and dishes, cleaning the counter, and returning everything to its original spot. This is a good habit to get into to keep the apothecary

running smoothly and keeping it sanitary. Deep cleaning and sanitization should be done based on how often it is used.

- **Inspect your supplies**: Occasionally, check the condition of your supplies. Look for wear and tear and check if any of them need to be replaced. Plan ahead for replacing much needed tools to help relieve a financial burden at the last minute.

Mary's Advice

Finish the journal or spreadsheet from the box in Chapter Eight (page 38) to know when you need to harvest herbs around you and what parts should be harvested at that time. From here you can determine what might need to be ordered instead.

- **Inventory**: An occasional inventory of your supplies and herbs is recommended. How often this is done is determined by how much the apothecary is used. This is important when you first start out and over the next few years to understand how much material you are using in the apothecary. This can affect how much you order and harvest over the following years. I personally inventory my herbs throughout the year because I use a lot of them. I use a spreadsheet with the herb, the parts, the lot numbers (if purchased), and the date harvested or purchased. I review this at least four times a year physically to check for any depletion of the herbs on the shelves along with the date of expiration of each. I determine from here if another order needs to be purchased or if more harvesting is needed. Supplies could include containers, menstrua (plural spelling of menstruum), oils, butters, essential oils, cheesecloth, lip balm containers, miscellaneous jars and bottles, or cleaning products.
- **Introduce new herbs or supplies**: As you learn more and gain more experience, you can add new herbs, herbal preparations, or supplies to the apothecary. You will slowly gain new herbal allies to use and possibly have new tools to make running the apothecary easier.

I think the easiest way to keep up with the needs of your apothecary is to be consistent in how you utilize it, clean it, and restock it so that it is functional at all times. You will appreciate this advice the more you use your apothecary.

PART EIGHT

Moving Forward

Chapter Twenty-Nine
Legalities Concerning Herbalism

As you continue practicing herbalism, there are some legal aspects that you need to be aware of in the United States of America. It matters what words you say, what you put on your labels, what words you use to advertise an herbal business, and what you say about your products. There are laws on both the state and federal levels that apply to herbalism, and it is best to check with your own state and the federal government for those laws. In Chapter Four (page 19), I let you know about laws pertaining to using the word "apothecary" in certain states. That's just one word. Let's break down some important concepts that should be uppermost in your mind at all times here in the United States.

The most important concept to understand is that herbalism is an unlicensed occupation unless you are an herbalist who is also licensed as a doctor. There are words and behaviors reserved for the licensed practitioner within the medical community, and they should never be replicated from someone who is unlicensed. Examples of words to be avoided at all costs are cure, treat, prescribe, diagnose, and patients. As far as behaviors go, an unlicensed herbalist will never cure, treat, offer prescriptions, or diagnose their clients. This pertains to all unlicensed herbalists, and these words and behaviors should be avoided to protect ourselves and the entire herbal community. This includes when you are teaching herbalism in person, on video, in written word, or on social media.

Another concept you need to understand is that herbs and herbal products are currently listed as dietary supplements. The FDA regulates the manufacturing process and all finished products produced for the market. According to their website, the FDA is responsible for protecting the public health by ensuring the safety, efficacy, and security of human and veterinary drugs, biological products, and medical devices, and by ensuring the safety of our nation's food supply, cosmetics, and products that emit radiation.[26] This means that a manufacturer or distributor of dietary supplements is responsible for evaluating the safety and labeling of their products before marketing to ensure that they meet all the requirements of the Federal Food, Drug, and Cosmetic Act as amended by DSHEA and FDA regulations.[27] Basically, there are a long list of regulations and laws that you need to be aware of prior to selling herbal products or bulk herbs if you decide to do that. You will need to read up on their Good Manufacturing Practice (GMP) Regulations. You can also take classes on GMPs from herbal experts, conferences, or organizations.

These FDA regulations prevent makers of dietary supplements from making any health claims on their products. This will automatically be considered a drug claim, and the product will no longer be considered a dietary supplement. You cannot mention any disease or symptom of a disease on the label. You also cannot make a claim about a product in the same space that you are selling it. Do not sell products on your website, social media, or in a written catalog where you also say what that herb's uses are. You cannot have testimonials about products either. There are additional laws and regulations that you should research before committing to the sale of herbal products to the public.

Teaching herbalism is a first amendment right that we have as US citizens. You can say anything or write anything about herbs as long as you are not also linking the sale of any product that contains that particular herb. If you speak about an herb and what it does while also promoting a product containing the herb, that is considered making a drug claim. If you are only making herbal preparations for yourself, your family, or your friends, you do not need to concern yourself with these laws; however, they do apply if you are charging money for the product to others. There are fine lines that need to be walked as an herbalist. Just be aware of those lines.

This chapter isn't meant to warn you away from seeing clients or from selling herbs and herbal preparations. It is meant to arm you with knowledge so that you, the general public, and the herbal community are all safe and protected. Ignorance is not an excuse when it comes to the government, and it is always best to be prepared before you make any decisions as you continue learning in herbalism.

Chapter Thirty
Next Steps

You have taken the first step into learning herbalism by reading this book, following the exercises, and creating your very own home apothecary. This book doesn't contain all the education needed to be proficient as an herbalist, nor does it talk about the more complex subjects taught in herbalism. I hope I have inspired you to continue learning, which will be necessary if you plan to do more with this knowledge in the future. I will offer additional steps you can take moving forward in your studies.

As I mentioned before, learning herbalism is a continued journey. I have been studying herbs for well over a decade, and I am still learning things I didn't know. I remember hearing Matthew Wood say that after he hit a decade as an herbalist, he thought he knew it all, but then found out he didn't. Another decade went by, and he was sure he knew it all, but then found out he didn't. Yet another decade went by in which he was now sure he knew everything he could know, but realized he didn't. I will never forget him telling this to us in the class. It was humbling and inspirational to me, and I personally continue to learn about other aspects or information in herbalism to accomplish the expansion of my own knowledge and practice.

Throughout this book, I have mentioned subjects that you can research more about, or take classes in. It is always beneficial to learn the history of herbalism and read some of the old materia medicas or herbals. I keep this knowledge with me as a comparison when learning some modern uses and new scientific data. You will also discover more details about how they deciphered energetics during that period of history, and you will be able to follow along with their thought processes with each health condition. You might also be enlightened to make historical herbal preparations that are not prevalent in today's society. There are some interesting ointments, wines, and other herbal blends that you can experiment with. Learn from both the past and the present.

Learning more details about botany can be beneficial moving forward to help further your identification skills. There are some highly skilled teachers and schools in that subject that you can learn from for pursuit of that information. I do not have a degree in botany. What I have learned, I learned from taking classes and from my own research. Seek those specialists out if that is a passion you wish to follow.

Skills in growing herbs from seed, transplanting those seedlings, planting established herbs, and caring for them are other steps you can take in the learning process. Not every herbalist wants to learn this skill or has a desire to grow herbs, but it is a good way of connecting more with the plants.

There are advanced medicine-making techniques that you can learn as well. I showed the folk method for ease of learning and less confusion as you start your journey, but there are more potent or quicker ways to make herbal medicine. Learn how mathematics is used to make herbal medicine and how that might differ from making them with the folk method. You can learn about percolations, double extractions, Soxhlet extractions, and enhance your formulation skills. In addition, plant chemistry and solubility are necessary subjects to understand more about why you are creating certain herbal preparations, what herbal preparations will give you the result you are looking for, and how much more potent each could become depending on how they are prepared.

Last, but not least, there are additional subjects to learn about if you are pursuing clinical herbalism as a career path. These subjects include anatomy and physiology, nutrition, biochemistry, and differential assessment skills. My advice is to learn as much as you can in the other subjects before beginning to learn about clinical herbalism. You need a complete understanding of herbalism with additional experience using it before you are able to move into clinical practice.

Where do you go from here? How should you go about it? These are questions that I hope I can answer with the following recommendations.

- **Learn one subject at a time**. It's tempting to take multiple classes or read multiple books about everything herbalism. The problem with doing this is it causes an individual to feel overwhelmed. Don't do that to yourself.

- **Practice using the herbs in this book until you feel proficient doing so**. This includes experiencing the effects or seeing the effects in action with each herb. It could also include growing, harvesting, and making additional herbal preparations with each one. Use this book for future reference.
- **Once you are ready, learn about another herb and gain experience using it**. Remember, it is not how many herbs you know, but how many you are proficient using.
- **Increase your identification skills**. Take hikes or walks around your area and document plants that you see. Find other herbalists offering plant walks. Take pictures, journal their locations and identifying characteristics, and see if you can identify the plant you saw.
- **Keep practicing**. Practice makes you gain confidence and valuable experience.
- **Continue journaling in herbalism**. Record the plants growing around you, keep a journal for harvesting times, document recipes with the amounts used and the results, document your experience with each herb. There are numerous things that you can add to your journals. These help with the retention of information, acts as a reference for yourself and possibly others, and keeps track of what works and what doesn't. This isn't mandatory in order to learn herbalism, but it helps you for the future.
- **Learn where to get reliable knowledge in herbalism**. In the next chapter, I will list some valuable resources for the continued study of herbalism. Be sure to review my research guidelines to help you navigate reliable information from other resources.
- **Use these resources**. Remember that it is best to learn from multiple reliable resources to get more clarification and better knowledge.

Chapter Thirty-One
Resources

This section of the book lists organizations, conferences, websites, suppliers, and other resources concerning herbalism that I am familiar with. These are some of the resources I have experience using and I feel comfortable recommending them. There are many more individual herbalists, schools, organizations, suppliers, and herbal conferences that you can find in your research, and some can come from the resources below. Review Chapter Two (page 9) if necessary for a review of my research guidelines.

Continued Education

- www.herbalistmentor.com: You can continue to this website to gain more education in herbalism. This is my website where I can offer you more resources of study such as:
  - Hands-on training and plant walk videos
  - Membership opportunities in furthering your education and gaining mentorship
  - Herb articles and my upcoming events
  - Links to Herbology Talk monthly meetups and its coordinating podcast
- **American Herbalists Guild**: This organization's mission is to promote clinical herbalism as a viable profession rooted in ethics, competency, diversity, and freedom of practice. The AHG supports access to herbal medicine for all and advocates excellence in herbal education. There is a Registered Herbalist membership and credential offered after a peer-reviewed application process that establishes a recognized level of expertise and commitment to the practice of herbalism. A list of these Registered Herbalists is located on their website along with those wishing to provide mentorship to others. Visit www.americanherbalistsguild.com and become a member for additional benefits in training. Receive

an extra $15 off membership with the code **MaryAHG15**. Here's some of what the AHG can offer:

- Legal and regulatory FAQs and Herbal Education FAQs
- A directory of herbal schools (schools pay to have their names listed)
- A list of books authored by Registered Herbalists
- A list of mentors available for mentorship
- Free webinars every month for the public
- Access to all recorded webinars and past symposium classes for members
- Webinar intensives offered to everyone with additional discounts for members
- Discounts to other businesses for members
- The *Journal of the American Herbalists Guild* available for members
- The opportunity to attend the Annual Symposium of the AHG available to all
- **American Botanical Council**: This organization's mission is to provide education using science-based and traditional information to promote responsible use of herbal medicine—serving the public researchers, educators, healthcare professionals, industry, and media. They educate on the safe and effective use of herbs and medicinal plants. Visit www.herbalgram.org. Students can benefit by becoming a member and receiving:
  - *HerbalGram*: quarterly journal of the American Botanical Council and HerbalEGram
  - Monographs and articles of herbs
  - Botanical Adulterants Prevention Program
  - Herbal News and Events
- **The United Plant Savers**: This organization's mission is to protect native medicinal plants, fungi, and their habitats while ensuring renewable populations for use by generations to come. Visit www.unitedplantsavers.org. They can offer students educational resources such as:
  - Species at-risk list
  - International Herb Symposium

- Partners in Education member list
- Events
- 360-acre botanical sanctuary located in Rutland, Ohio
- *Journal of Medicinal Plant Conservation*
- **HerbRally**: This website began with herbalism events but has evolved into so much more. HerbRally aims to provide you with a premier resource for discovering herbal education in all of its beautiful forms. Visit www.herbrally.com. Educational opportunities include:
  - HerbRally Podcast
  - Herbal events and schools
  - Monographs, YouTube, and a blog
  - Schoolhouse membership opportunity
- **Plant Healer**: Hedgewise Academy of Folk Herbalism offers multiple resources for the beginner herbalist concentrating on hedgewise wisdom and practical skills for an empowered, vitally effective, and delight-filled herbalism. Visit www.planthealer.org. They offer students in herbalism:
  - A bookstore
  - An opportunity to sign up for Herbaria monthly
  - An opportunity to purchase *Plant Healer Quarterly* magazine
  - Good Medicine Confluence gathering annually
- **Great Lakes Herb Faire**: Located at Cedar Lake Outdoor Center in Chelsea, Michigan, annually in September, this conference is the closest to me and includes many great opportunities to learn from experienced herbalists from many different facets of life. Visit www.greatlakesherbfaire.org.
- **The Herbarium**: A vibrant virtual archive of herbal resources. This is a convenient and affordable online library that's packed with trustworthy herbal resources and reference materials. Visit www.theherbalacademy.com. They offer:
  - Plant monographs
  - Herbal intensives
  - Herbal articles

- Free media downloads
- Educational videos and podcasts
- Herbal book recommendations

Apothecary Suppliers

- **Mountain Rose Herbs**: www.mountainroseherbs.com
- **Zack Woods Herb Farm**: zachwoodsherbs.com
- **Frontier Co-op**: www.frontiercoop.com
- **Mushroom Harvest**: www.mushroomharvest.com
- **Pacific Botanicals**: www.pacificbotanicals.com
- **Penn Herb Company**: www.pennherb.com
- **Starwest Botanicals**: www.starwest-botanicals.com
- **Strictly Medicinal Herbs**: www.strictlymedicinalseeds.com
- **Companion Plants**: www.companionplants.com
- **Oshala Farm**: www.oshalafarm.com
- **Mulberry Creek Herbs**: www.mulberrycreek.com
- **Specialty Bottles**: www.specialtybottle.com

Research your own area for additional resources such as farmers, organic herb growers, or other herbalists that you might be able to purchase herbs from. Sometimes other herbalists will barter for something they don't have. The bartering system is still alive and well today! You can also find more resources at the American Herbalists Guild website that are offering discounts for their members.

Glossary

Adaptogen: A medicinal property that supports the body's immune system while helping the body deal with stress and its many effects.

Aerial part: When harvesting herbs, this refers to all of the parts above the ground.

Alterative: Helps to correct impure conditions of the blood by helping to support elimination channels of the body.

Amphoteric: The capability of an herb to have opposing actions in order to balance or normalize an organ or system in the body.

Analgesic: A medicinal property taken internally to relieve pain.

Annual: The completion of a plant's life cycle in one year.

Anodyne: A medicinal property taken externally to relieve pain.

Anthelmintic: A medicinal property used to destroy or expel worms.

Antifungal: A medicinal property that inhibits or destroys the growth of fungus.

Anti-inflammatory: A medicinal property that prevents or reduces inflammation—also referred to as antiphlogistic.

Antilithic: A medicinal property that prevents the formation of urinary calculi (stones) and can help in their removal.

Antimicrobial: This medicinal property helps to resist, deter, or kill microorganisms.

Antioxidant: This refers to the prevention of oxidative stress or damage from oxidation.

Antiphlogistic: This property refers to the prevention or reduction of inflammation, or in other words, anti-inflammatory.

Antiproliferative: Suppresses malignant cell growth.

Antiseptic: This medicinal property will help to prevent or counteract infection or the decaying of cells.

Antispasmodic: A medicinal property that will relax contracted muscular tissue (or spasms).

Anxiolytic: A medicinal property that reduces anxiety.

Aperient: A medicinal property of an herb that has a mild laxative action without the usual griping pain and stimulates the appetite and digestion.

Aphrodisiac: A medicinal property that enhances sexual desire/the ability to perform the act along with increasing pleasure.

Apothecary: A person or place that prepared and supplied medicine. An archaic term used before the modern pharmacist or modern medicine.

Aromatherapy: The practice of using aroma as a complementary health approach.

Aromatics: Herbs with a strong fragrance or taste that tend to support the digestive, respiratory, and nervous systems.

Astringent: A medicinal property that tightens tissue when it is relaxed, weak, or injured.

Atony: A structural tissue state referring to lack of tone.

Atrophy: A tissue state referring to the lack of fluids in the body contributing to the wasting away of organs or cells.

Axillary bud: A bud located at the axil of a leaf capable of producing a branch or flower cluster.

Bark: Protective outer sheath of a tree or woody shrub.

Biennial: Life cycle of a plant is completed in two years.

Bitters: Bitter tasting herbs extracted in alcohol specifically used for digestive purposes.

Bolus: An herbal mixture of powdered herbs and melted coconut oil or cocoa butter shaped and inserted into an orifice.

Botany: The study and classification of plants.

Carminative: The medicinal property that relieves and dispels flatulence in the gastrointestinal tract.

Catalyst: Herb added to a formula for enhancement, absorption, and direction of the medicine.

Cathartic: This medicinal property produces purgative actions in the intestinal tract.

Cell proliferant: This medicinal property repairs the cells in the body.

Cholagogue: This medicinal property stimulates bile production and encourages release in the liver and gallbladder.

Cold infusion: An herb steeped in cold water for a length of time.

Concentrated preparation: A stronger preparation you get by simmering an infusion or decoction to reduce the volume.

Constituent: Individual and active ingredients that make up the whole plant producing medicinal benefits.

Constitutions: The energetics of a person (human energetics).

Constriction state: This structural tissue state refers to body tissue being too tense.

Contraindications: A condition or symptom that makes a remedy unsuitable or dangerous for that individual.

Cream: A thick moisturizing mixture using oil and water combined.

Decoction: A water extract with an extended period of heating. Used for material such as roots or bark that need an extension of heat to extract the medicine.

Demulcent: A medicinal property that soothes irritated tissue internally.

Deobstruent: A medicinal property that removes obstructions in the body that prevent the flow of fluid or secretions.

Depression: Another term referring to a cold tissue state in which there is depressed or slow activity.

Depurant: Having a purifying or detoxifying action.

Dermal limits: This is the maximum percentage of essential oil allowed in a product.

Diaphoretic: A medicinal property that increases perspiration for either the reduction of fever or for help in elimination.

Digestive: A medicinal property that supports and aids the digestive system.

Diuretic: This medicinal property increases the secretion and flow of urine.

Doctrine of Signatures: A theory where the plant's physical appearance resembles the therapeutic value in the body.

Dose: A quantity of medicine taken.

Douche: This application uses an herbal infusion or decoction and is inserted into the vagina using a fountain syringe.

Drop dosing: Uses very small amounts of an herb medicinally to balance the body.

Electuaries: When powdered herbs are mixed with something sweet for consumption.

Elixir: A sweetened tincture.

Emetic: This medicinal property induces vomiting.

Emmenagogue: This medicinal property regulates or induces menstruation.

Emollient: This medicinal property soothes tissue externally.

Enema: This application uses an herbal infusion or decoction and is inserted into the anus.

Energetics: Patterns are both observed and utilized to balance an individual and their health conditions with an herb(s).

Errhine: Increases nasal secretions from sinus cavities.

Essential oils: Isolated and condensed volatile oils (aroma component) of an herb and are used in aromatherapy.

Excitation: Heated tissue state.

Expectorant: Promotes the discharge of mucus from the lungs.

Extract: The process of pulling out constituents from herbs into a menstruum.

Febrifuge: Reduces fever.

Flower: Seed bearing part of a plant.

Flower essence: Preparation used to work on the emotional well-being of individuals.

Fomentation: Moist therapy using an infusion or decoction of herbs.

Four qualities: Energetic philosophy consisting of the temperature and action of an herb.

Fruit: Ripened ovary of a plant containing seeds.

Galactagogue: Increases the flow of milk production.

Girdling: Making a cut around the trunk of a tree.

Glycerite: Extract using vegetable glycerin.

Harvesting: Collecting parts of a plant to use for medicine.

Hemagogue: Promotes the flow of blood.

Hemostatic: Stops or controls bleeding, or antihemorrhagic.

Hepatic: In relation to the liver.

Herb: Herbaceous plant defined as a seed-bearing plant without a woody stem that dies back after flowering (annual, perennial, or biennial).

Herbal bath: Soaking in a water extraction of herb(s).

Herbal extract: Herbal preparation using a liquid to extract constituents from an herb(s).

Herbal preparation: Herbal medicine using multiple methods of extraction.

Herbalism: The practice of using herbal medicine.

Herbology: The study of using plants as medicine.

Homeopathy: Natural substances utilized with the "like curing like" philosophy in minute doses.

Homeostasis: Self-regulation process in the body.

Hull: Outer covering of a seed or fruit.

Human energetics: Patterns observed in an individual and their health conditions.

Hypertensive: Raises blood pressure.

Hypotensive: Lowers blood pressure.

Indications: A sign indicating the best herb to choose.

Interactions: How an herb can affect the action of a pharmaceutical drug.

Lanceolate leaf: Narrow-shaped leaf with the end coming to a point.

Lactifuge: Reduces milk flow.

Leaves: Flat structure attached to the stem or stalk of a plant.

Liniment: An external use of an extract using alcohol, witch hazel, or vinegar.

Lithotriptic: Dissolves kidney or bladder stones.

Lotion: Liquid used externally to moisturize containing water and oil.

Low-dose botanical: An herb that should only be taken in drop doses.

Lymphatic: A medicinal property stimulating the lymphatic system.

Macerating: The act of extracting herbs in liquid for a period of time.

Maceration: The process of extracting herbs in a liquid for a period of time.

Marc: The herb macerating in liquid.

Maximum dosing: Using the highest dose of an herb allowed to create an action.

Medicinal properties: How an herb acts with the body. Interchangeable term with medicinal actions.

Menstruum: The liquid used in the extraction process.

Mucilaginous: Contains mucilage (gel-like polysaccharide substance in plants).

Nephritic: In relation to the kidneys.

Nervine: Supports the nervous system. These can be sub-categorized as relaxing, stimulating, or as a tonic to the nervous system.

Nootropic: Improves cognitive function and memory.

Nutritive: Containing many nutrients.

Nuts: Hardened fruit from a tree or plant with a shell.

Oil: A base oil infused with herbs.

Ointment: Herbal infused oil with beeswax to harden it.

Organoleptic: An herb's effect determined by the senses.

Oxymel: Herbal preparation using vinegar and honey.

Parturient: Stimulates uterine contractions to hasten childbirth.

Pectoral: Healing to the lungs.

Perennial: Plant that continues to grow year after year for several years.

Plant energetics: Term referring to descriptive patterns of plants consisting of qualities and tastes.

Plaster: An external application of powdered or dried plant material moistened and placed onto a cloth and secured with a plastic wrap.

Poultice: Fresh moistened herbs applied directly to the skin.

Pulse dosing: dosing requiring breaks in ingesting the herb.

Purgative: Causes evacuation of bowels usually with griping pain. Strong laxative.

Refrigerant: Cools body temperature and relieves thirst.

Relaxant: Relieves tension.

Resin: Thick, sticky substance obtained from the gum or sap of trees.

Root: Underground part of plant supplying nutrients and water.

Rubefacient: Stimulates capillary dilation and skin redness upon external application.

Salve: An ointment.

Sap: Thin, sugary substance produced by trees.

Sedative: Having a tranquilizing effect.

Shelf expectancy: Length of time a product is expected to be viable.

Sialagogue: Promotes secretion and flow of saliva.

Simple: Single herb used in medicine rather than a formula of multiple herbs.

Stagnation: Not flowing or moving.

Standard dose: A dosing philosophy used in herbalism that provides adequate medicinal actions.

Standardization: Process of developing standards in medicine.

Steam: The delivery of medicinal properties through steam.

Steam distillation: Process of extracting and condensing volatile oils from a plant.

Stimulant: Increases body function.

Stomachic: Stimulates and tonifies the stomach.

Succus: The use of plant juice in an herbal preparation.

Sustainability: Avoidance of depleting our natural resources and contributing to the balance of the ecosystem for future generations.

Syrup: An infusion or decoction with added equal amounts of honey.

Taeniafuge: Expels a tapeworm.

Taenicide: Kills a tapeworm.

Tincture: An extract using alcohol as the menstruum.

Tisane: An extract using water as the menstruum.

Tissue states: A form of energetics describing the state of tissue in a body.

Tonic: Strengthening and increases tone.

Trophorestorative: Rebuilding, restorative, and nourishing.

Urtication: The practice of using stinging nettle to reduce inflammation by flogging oneself with the stinging leaves.

Vermicide: Kills worms.

Vermifuge: Expels worms.

Vinegar: An extract using vinegar as the menstruum.

Volatile oil: The aromatic compounds of a plant.

Vulnerary: Promoting healing of wounds.

Warm infusion: Another name for a tisane or warm extraction of plants using water.

Directory of Herbal Formulas and Remedies

Endnotes

1. Wood, Matthew, *The Book of Herbal Wisdom*, 1997, North Atlantic Books, Berkeley, California, pp. 31, 47.

2. World Health Organization, "Safety issues in the preparation of homeopathic medicines," 2009, WHO Press, Switzerland, pg. ix.

3. Bach, Edward; Wheeler, F.J.; Dr. Edward Back Centre, *The Bach Flower Remedies*, 1997, The C.W. Daniel Company Ltd., Saffron Walden, Essex, England, pg. ix.

4. "Medieval Occupations and Jobs: Apothecary. History of apothecary and their products," accessed June 2, 2022, https://medievalbritain.com/type /medieval-life/occupations/medieval-apothecary/.

5. "The Role of an Apothecary in the Middle Ages: The work of healers in Medieval times," accessed June 4, 2022, https://worldhistory.us/medieval -history/the-role-of-an-apothecary-in-the-middle-ages-the-work-of-healers -in-medieval-times.php.

6. Ohio Revised Code/Title 47 Occupations-Professions Chapter 4729, Pharmacists Dangerous Drugs Section 4729.36 (Advertisements), 1998.

7. Johnson, Thomas, Gerard, John, *The Generall Historie of Plantes: Selections from the 1633 Enlarged and Amended Edition Gerard's Herbal*, 2008 (1633), Velluminous Press, pg. 352.

8. Hare, Hobart Amory, et al., *National Standard Dispensatory*, 1905, Lea Brothers & Co., Philadelphia and New York, pg. 963.

9. Brown, O. Phelps, *The Complete Herbalist*, 1875, Self-published, Jersey City, New Jersey, pp. 41, 151.

10. Moacă EA, Farcaş C, Ghiţu A, et al. "A Comparative Study of *Melissa officinalis* Leaves and Stems Ethanolic Extracts in terms of Antioxidant, Cytotoxic, and Antiproliferative Potential." *Evid Based Complement Alternat Med.* 2018;2018:7860456. Published 2018 May 16. doi:10.1155/2018/7860456.

11. Cech, Richo, *Making Plant Medicine*, Fourth Edition, 2016, Herbal Reads, Williams, Oregon, pg. 264.

12. Culpeper, Nicholas, *Culpeper's Complete Herbal, and English Physician*, 1813, J. Tregortha, Burslem.

13. Oberlin College, Western Reserve Land Conservancy Firelands, Chapter, *Living in the Vermilion River Watershed*, 2008, POV Communications, Chardon, Ohio, pg. 2.

14. Wood, Matthew, *The Earthwise Herbal: A Complete Guide to the New World Medicinal Plants*, 2009, North Atlantic Books, Berkeley, California, pp. 208, 264, 351.

15. Flint, Margi, *The Practicing Herbalist*, 2013, Earthsong Press, Marblehead, Massachusetts, pg. 268.

16. Oladeji OS, Oyebamiji AK. "*Stellaria media* (L.) Vill.—A plant with immense therapeutic potentials: phytochemistry and pharmacology." *Heliyon*. 2020;6(6):e04150. Published 2020 Jun 7. doi:10.1016/j.heliyon.2020.e04150.

17. Stickel F, Seitz HK. "The efficacy and safety of comfrey." *Public Health Nutr*. 2000;3(4A):501-508. doi:10.1017/s1368980000000586.

18. Awang, Dennis V.C., "Comfrey update" Summer 1991. *American Botanical Council Herbalgram*, Issue 25, pp. 20–23.

19. Zhai Z, Liu Y, Wu L, et al. "Enhancement of innate and adaptive immune functions by multiple Echinacea species." *J Med Food*. 2007;10(3):423–434. doi:10.1089/jmf.2006.257.

20. Christopher, John R., *School of Natural Healing: Centennial Edition*, 2009, Christopher Publications, Springville, Utah, pp. 53, 90, 328.

21. Tassell MC, Kingston R, Gilroy D, Lehane M, Furey A. Hawthorn, "(Crataegus spp.) in the treatment of cardiovascular disease." *Pharmacogn Rev*. 2010 Jan;4(7):32–41. doi: 10.4103/0973-7847.65324. PMID: 22228939; PMCID: PMC3249900.

22. Ransome, Hilda, *The Sacred Bee in Ancient Times and Folklore*, 2004, Dover Publications, Mineola, New York, pp. 94, 96.

23. Jahanban-Esfahlan A, Modaeinama S, Abasi M, Abbasi MM, Jahanban-Esfahlan R. "Anti Proliferative Properties of *Melissa officinalis* in Different Human Cancer Cells." *Asian Pac J Cancer Prev*. 2015;16(14):5703–5707. doi:10.7314/apjcp.2015.16.14.5703.

24. Ao Z, Chan M, Ouyang MJ, et al. "Identification and evaluation of the inhibitory effect of *Prunella vulgaris* extract on SARS-coronavirus 2 virus entry." *PLoS One*. 2021;16(6):e0251649. Published 2021 Jun 9. doi:10.1371/journal.pone.0251649.

25. Pederson, Mark, *Nutritional Herbology: A Reference Guide to Herbs*, 2010, Whitman Publications, Warsaw, Indiana, pp. 145, 177.

26. US Food and Drug Administration, "What We Do," FDA Mission, November 11, 2022, https://fda.gov/about-fda/what-we-do.

27. US Food and Drug Administration, "Dietary Supplements," November 11, 2022, https://www.fda.gov/food/dietary-supplements.

Index